DOCTOR DOCK

Doctor Dock

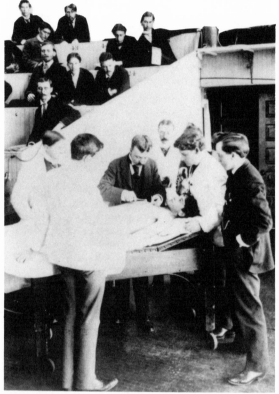

TEACHING AND LEARNING MEDICINE
AT THE TURN OF THE CENTURY
Horace W. Davenport

RUTGERS UNIVERSITY PRESS   New Brunswick and London

Library of Congress Cataloging-in-Publication Data

Davenport, Horace Willard, 1912–
Doctor Dock.

1. Medical education—Michigan—History—20th
century.   2. Diagnosis—Study and teaching—Michigan—
History—20th century.   3. Dock, George, 1860–
4. University of Michigan.   Medical Dept.   I. Title.
[DNLM: 1. Dock, George, 1860–   .   2. University of
Michigan.   Medical Dept.   3. Education, Medical—
biography.   4. Education, Medical—history—Michigan.
5. Teaching—methods.   WZ 100 D637D]
R746.M45D38   1987   610'.7'1177435   86-17842
ISBN 0-8135-1190-9

British CIP information available.

For I.C.D.

Contents

Illustrations

Preface

GEORGE DOCK'S *CLINICAL NOTES* DEMONSTRATE HOW MEDICINE
was practiced and taught by a good man in a good medical school at the beginning of the twentieth century.

The *Clinical Notes* are the typed transcript of the stenographic record of everything that was said in twice-weekly diagnostic clinics Dock conducted for
the fourth-year medical students at the University of Michigan in the academic
years 1899–1900 through 1907–1908. There is no transcript for the year
1902–1903. The transcript is typed double spaced on 8-½-by-11-inch paper of
good quality, and it is bound in sixteen volumes, two for each year.

The typist sometimes inserted (couldn't hear.), but often she left a blank or
typed (I thought he said [so-and-so]). Sometimes but not usually Dock filled the
blank in pencil. Whether or not he did, I have filled it when I understood or
guessed what was omitted. When I did not understand, I have either left the
blank or filled it with a conjecture in square brackets. There are omissions, particularly in the earlier volumes, that cannot be filled. For example, at the end of
the transcript for November 3, 1899, Dock wrote: "Evidently much left out here
—as to Banti—reason for operating, &c." Another gap occurs when Dock was
sick or out of town. Then the clinic was conducted by whomever was his current
first assistant, James Arneill, Roger Morris, Hugo Freund or Frank Smithies. I
have not used the transcripts of those clinics except once to quote James Arneill.

I have not altered the sentence structure, and I have retained the typist's
punctuation, with the exception of inserting omitted question marks, for they
convey the flavor of Dock's speech. Likewise, in the quoted transcripts I have retained spelling that reflects the usage of the day. A swollen thyroid gland is always a *goitre*. The sensation of labored breathing is sometimes *dyspnoea* and
sometimes *dyspnea*. The pigment of the erythrocytes is indifferently spelled *hae-
moglobin* or *hemoglobin*. In early transcripts the *oe* and *ae* are typed with a
ligature.

The typist had trouble with technical words, and in October of 1903 the
spelling was particularly fanciful. In a patient with suspected typhoid fever the
venal test was negative, and a patient with *syonosis* had *adema* of the ankles.

xi

This was done by a new typist, Miss O. Dock must have had a frank talk with the bewildered girl, for the spelling soon improved and remained good as Miss O. typed the rest of the transcripts through 1907–1908. Dock sometimes corrected the spelling in pencil in an almost illegible hand, but often he did not. At the end of 1904 *haemoplegia* remained uncorrected. When I quote the text I have silently corrected such trivial misspellings.

I have altered the text in two ways:

1. Dock sometimes gave an impromptu lecture on various topics—home treatment of tuberculosis, how to give a hypodermic injection, the technique and effectiveness of vaccination and the like. The lectures were usually discursive. I have eliminated irrelevant parts, retaining what I believe to have been the central message. When Dock gave a similar lecture another year, I may have added some of its content to the first. Thus, what I present in a single paragraph may be derived from ten or more pages of transcript.

2. Over the years Dock demonstrated more than a hundred patients with tuberculosis and a like number with valvular heart disease or typhoid fever. Although there was only one patient with plague, there were thirty with thyroid disease. It would be intolerably tedious to quote independently a sufficient number of transcripts to illustrate the full range of Dock's teaching and practice. Instead, I have drawn quotations from many transcripts and conflated them to show how Dock dealt with each medical problem.

This is not a Ph.D. dissertation, and I have not pedantically identified with footnotes all the dates on which Dock, the students, and the patients said what I quote. I cite a date only when it illuminates the text. For example, I say that the first record of instrumental measurement of blood pressure was made on October 27, 1903. I have condensed the text and rearranged its parts, but I have added nothing. The casual reader can be certain that everything I attribute to the speakers occurs someplace in those more than 6,800 pages of transcript. In 1945 dock deposited his *Clinical Notes* in the Michigan Historical Collections, and they are now preserved in the Bentley Historical Library on the north campus of the University of Michigan in Ann Arbor. The scholar or the skeptic can compare the *Clinical Notes* with an annotated copy of this book that I have also deposited in the Bentley Historical Library.

I have presented George Dock's medicine strictly in terms of contemporary knowledge. I have identified books and journal articles referred to by Dock, and when necessary I have explained the reference. On occasion I have compared Dock's teaching with that of persons he knew or could have known. Examples are his Michigan colleague Arthur Robertson Cushny and James Mackenzie of Burnley and London. Because Dock was a protégé of William Osler and practiced and taught very much in the Osler manner, I have compared what Dock said with what Osler wrote in the third (1898) and sixth (1906) editions of *The*

Principles and Practice of Medicine. That textbook was studied by Dock's students. The reader, if he thinks the practice and teaching of medicine have vastly improved since Dock's time, can judge Dock in the light of knowledge accumulated after 1908, but I have not done so.

H.W.D.

Acknowledgments

MY GREATEST DEBT IS TO GEORGE DOCK FOR LEAVING BEHIND A document from which I could assemble a partial portrait of Dock himself as well as an account of turn-of-the-century medicine. It has been a great pleasure to make Dock's acquaintance, and I am especially grateful to him for giving me the opportunity to write the only book on the history of medicine that is intentionally amusing.

—I thank George Dock's son, William Dock, and his grandson, Donald Dock, for permission to quote the *Clinical Notes*.

—I thank the staff of the Michigan Historical Collections, the Bentley Historical Library, and in particular John Wimsatt, for help. The Department of Pathology of the University of Michigan Medical School made autopsy records readily available.

Saul Jarcho and L. J. Bruce-Chwatt courteously answered my questions during my futile search for printed evidence of Dock's failure to identify mosquitoes as the vector of malaria.

Friday, May 12th, 1905.

PATIENTS: Carpenter (Hector), Mrs. Gibson (G. H. Lewis).

SECTION: Signor, Taylor, Thomas, Urquhart, Van den Berg.

Dr. We can pick out those who are neither lovers of music or base ball.

CARPENTER: Dr. Van den Berg, what do you think of this man? S. He looks sick. Dr. How does he look sick? S. His cheeks are slightly flushed and his eyes look rather bad. Dr, And what else? S. He is listless. Dr. What else do you notice about him? I think there is another thing that you ought to see. You have to be able to see it easily because when you see it at home it is usually in the alcove if there is an alcove about the house and the alcove is usually darkened so as to keep the air out as well as the light. S. I think there is cyanosis. Dr. That is the idea. There is cyanosis in his nose and it seems to me a little in his ears and lips and if we look at his hands we see a little in his nails, don't we? Otherwise there isn't anything so very striking about all that we can see of him now, is there? Let's see his tongue. Do you think there is anything abnormal about it? S. Why the terminal papillæ show very plainly. Dr. What else is there about it? How about the coating? He has a scanty but rather striking looking coat; that is the sort of a tongue that

FIGURE 1. A typical page of the transcript of the stenographic record of George Dock's teaching. The comment about music refers to the fact that the third concert of the May Festival was given that afternoon. At the same time Michigan beat Wisconsin 7 to 4 in baseball.

GEORGE DOCK AND THE MEDICAL SCHOOL

1.

IN THE ACADEMIC YEAR 1899–1900
and for many years thereafter, fourth-year medical students in the Department of Medicine and Surgery of the University of Michigan attended a medical diagnostic clinic every Tuesday and Friday afternoon in term time. George Dock, A.M., M.D., professor of theory and practice of medicine and clinical medicine, conducted the clinics. From at least October 3, 1899, he had a secretary make a shorthand record of everything that was said by Dock himself, the students, and the patients, and this practice continued until two weeks before Dock left Michigan for Tulane University in the summer of 1908. The secretary's typed transcript of those notes taken in eight of those years fills sixteen volumes totaling more than 6,800 pages. This book is a distillation, based upon those *Clinical Notes*, of what happened in the clinics.

A Characteristic Page

Here is a characteristic page:

Tuesday, March 5th, 1907.
PATIENTS: Mrs. Naveaux (Jones), Mrs. Coleman (McDonald), Mrs. Miller (McLellan).

SECTION: Miss Berry, Miss Humphrey, Culver, Fleumer, Grant, Gregory.

MRS. COLEMAN: Dr. Miss Berry, have you seen this lady before? What do you think about her. S. (Couldn't hear.) Dr. Why? S. She has dyspnoea; her mouth is drawn. Dr. What else do you see, Miss Humphrey? S. Her lips look purple but then— Dr. She is not

1

distinctly cyanotic, though, is she? What else do you see? S. She has some pulsation in her neck. Dr. And what else? S. A marked dyspnoea. Dr. What is the character of her dyspnoea? Yes, the expiration is prolonged and labored. What else? Yes, there is an epigastric pulsation. What do you suppose is the matter with her. S. I suppose there is some heart lesion. Dr. What would you do next in order to see? S. I would percuss the heart and auscult. Dr. Suppose you go ahead and examine the heart. S. There is a strong apex beat. Dr. Can you localize it? Where? S. It is in the nipple line. Dr. Where is the upper border? Do you think that it is dull there? Where is the absolute dulness? Suppose you go a little bit lower and see what you get. Where is the beginning of absolute dulness? Why do you have such a fear of going lower down? Where is the left side? That gives you the lower border, doesn't it? Now how are you going to get the left side? You can't percuss through the mammary gland, . . .

The names in parentheses are those of the students responsible for the patients on the ward. The students in the section are those Dock was taking on ward rounds in the morning and who were called upon to examine the patients used for demonstration.

George Dock

George Dock was born in Hopewell, Pennsylvania, on April 1, 1860, and he graduated A.B. from the University of Pennsylvania in 1881. The *Clinical Notes* show that he had a sound liberal education. His English was good; he often used the subjuctive mood; and he chose his words carefully. An occasional slip such as *enervated* for *innervated* or *effect* for *affect* can be blamed on the typist rather than Dock. Dock read Latin, and he insisted that students use it correctly. A passage like this occurs twice in the *Clinical Notes*:

DOCK: Lineae albicanta—that is another thing I found on examination papers and I can't understand it. What does albicans mean?

STUDENT: White.

DOCK: But how about lineae, what is the gender of lineae? Where did you get your Latin?

STUDENT: I got it after I came here.

DOCK: You are a lucky man. Would you call it albicanta then? Lineae is what gender?

STUDENT: Feminine.

DOCK: Then the adjective won't be albicanta. [The marks on the patient's skin] look like lineae albicantes; and indicate that the woman has been pregnant or had a very large abdominal tumor, though tumors rarely cause such lines.

Dock pronounced *abdomen* as *abdomen*, and he corrected a student who said *abdómen*. Once a student mocked him by saying: "The most distinctive thing is that in his abdomen or abdómen [there is a large tumor mass]." There is no indication how Dock pronounced *duodenum*, but we can hope it was not the surgeon's favorite *duwawdnum*.

Dock completed Pennsylvania's three-year medical course in 1884. While he was a medical student, Pennsylvania, like Michigan, was slowly transforming itself. Its dominating figure was William Pepper, called by Dock an acute diagnostician and an eloquent lecturer. Pepper was so eloquent, in fact, that when lecturing on pernicious anemia he could pass off the color of a jaundiced patient for that of an anemic one. Dock was taught medicine almost entirely by lecture or by demonstration clinics. He told Michigan medical students that "I remember, for example, if an interesting patient was brought into the clinic, and enterprising students would afterwards waylay him and by means of main strength or a small bribe get him to submit to an examination, but men got the title of doctor of medicine, with many elaborations in Latin, without having to handle a sick man."

In those days almost every student went immediately into practice after receiving such a diploma, but Dock interned for a year at St. Mary's, a Catholic hospital in an industrial part of Philadelphia. Many of the nurses were German nuns, and Dock learned German from them so that he would be prepared when, in the next two years, he studied in Germany and Austria with Krehl, Romberg, Virchow, Zemann, Paltauf and Weigert. Later he could speak German with patients in Ann Arbor, and Miss O. correctly transcribed what he said. Sometimes Dock told Michigan students one or another experience at St. Mary's or in Europe, and some of those stories will be quoted in their place.

In 1884 a retirement on Pennsylvania's faculty left the chair of clinical medicine vacant, and Pennsylvania acquired William Osler to fill it. Osler always maintained a private consulting practice, but he did not disappear from the school after lecturing, the way William Pepper did. Instead, he took students onto the wards of the University Hospital and of Old Blockley and into the autopsy room. Osler and John Herr Musser each contributed $50 to fit up a laboratory for clinical chemistry under a lecture theater, and when George Dock returned from Europe in 1887 he was put in charge of the laboratory. Dock formed a lasting friendship with Osler, and, following Osler's example, he became a competent pathologist and a more than competent clinician. When he was established at Michigan, Dock took "braindusting" trips to Europe with Osler, and together they made a pious visit to Boerhaave's house. Dock accompanied Osler to sales at Sotheby's, and like Osler he collected rare medical books and became something of a historian of medicine.[1]

Michigan at the Time of George Dock's Recruitment

In 1850, when Michigan's Department of Medicine and Surgery began to teach, it differed from other American medical schools in that it was an integral part of the university.[2] Two of its five professors were already members of the university faculty, Silas Douglass in chemistry and Abram Sager in botany. Students did not buy tickets for lectures, for the professors were paid salaries by the university. Two strong-minded and progressive university presidents, Henry P. Tappan (1852–1863) and James B. Angell (1871–1909), often presided at medical faculty meetings, and if they did not initiate they always approved actions affecting the medical school.

At first the curriculum consisted of a series of lectures lasting from October to April, and students were required to attend the series twice. Students were also expected to submit a thesis on the order of a term paper and to complete a three-year apprenticeship with a "respectable physician." From 1854 until his death in 1887, Alonzo B. Palmer was a dominating figure on the medical faculty as professor of medicine and pathology and then as dean. He was a clinician of the old school, but he participated in the evolution of the school. When Palmer was chairman of the American Medical Association's Committee on Medical Education, he agreed that admission requirements should be raised, that a graded and lengthened course should be introduced, that examinations should be more rigorous and that students should have "not less than two years of clinical instruction within the wards of a well-regulated hospital." All were accomplished at Michigan when George Dock arrived in 1891.

In 1856 the university completed the chemical laboratory, the first building in an American university to be devoted entirely to chemistry. Because Silas Douglass was superintendent of buildings and grounds as well as professor of chemistry in the medical school, he placed the building immediately adjacent to the medical building. The chemical laboratory remained administratively under the medical school until after George Dock had left Michigan. There medical students did laboratory work on urinalysis, toxicology and physiological chemistry, along with students in the university's literary and engineering departments. Victor Clarence Vaughan came to Michigan in 1874 to study chemistry in the chemical laboratory because many of the textbooks he had used in backwoods colleges in Missouri had been written by members of the Michigan faculty. He obtained a Ph.D. in chemistry and zoology in 1876, and in the same year he was appointed to teach physiological chemistry. Because chemistry was part of the medical school, Vaughan studied medicine, obtaining his M.D. in 1878. Vaughan began to teach bacteriology in 1881, although he had no formal training in the subject. In 1888 he and his protégé Frederick G. Novy spent the summer learning bacteriological techniques in Robert Koch's Berlin institute. When they returned to Ann Arbor they established a hygienic laboratory in the newly-constructed hygiene and physics building. In addition to providing a rigorous and modern course in bacteriology for medical students, Vaughan made the hygienic laboratory a school of public health in everything but name. Until the state laboratories were opened in Lansing many years later, all analyses for the state were done on the campus of the university, and engineers were taught medicine at the same time physicians were taught sanitary engineering.

When the medical faculty in 1880 began to look for a qualified physiologist, Vaughan took the initiative. He brought Henry Sewall, a student of Newell Martin, Carl Ludwig, Willi Kühne and J. N. Langley, to Ann Arbor as a candidate. Although Palmer preferred Charles Sedgwick Minot, Vaughan saw that Sewall was elected in 1881, and the next year Sewall began a full course in physiology for medical students. He cooperated with Vaughan in teaching bacteriology as well.

When Dean Palmer died in 1887, the medical faculty elected Corydon La Ford, its oldest member, dean, but Ford left all the dean's powers in Vaughan's hands. Vaughan was formally appointed dean in 1891, and he directed the school from 1888 until he retired in 1921.

Vaughan's first and major task was recruitment of faculty, and in that he was helped by a regent, Hermann Kiefer. Kiefer had been trained in Germany, but because he had participated in the Revolutions of 1848 and 1849 he had to flee to the United States. He attained a leading position in both Michigan medicine and the Republican party, but he gave up practice in 1891 to devote full time to the affairs of the medical school. Together Vaughan and Kiefer traveled throughout the country, looking for faculty, and in 1891, after some fumbling, they found George Dock.[3]

George Dock's Colleagues:
The Basic Scientists

Vaughan and Novy were responsible for teaching and research in physiological chemistry as well as bacteriology throughout Dock's time at Michigan. Textbooks, laboratory manuals and examination questions they wrote show that their teaching was thorough and up-to-date. The laboratory work was particularly rigorous, and Novy kept students in the laboratory well past scheduled hours by giving an examination at the end of each session. Dock's *Clinical Notes* contain a comment that the ambition of every student upon graduation was to kill Dr. Novy. Vaughan and Novy each attained enough distinction in research to be elected to the National Academy of Sciences, though one suspects that Vaughan's election was more a reward for his numerous administrative services than for his research accomplishments.

Henry Sewall had to resign in 1889 on account of his tuberculosis. Vaughan replaced him with William Henry Howell, another Johns Hopkins man. While he was in Ann Arbor, Howell completed his work on hematopoiesis, in which he identified what are known as the Howell-Jolly bodies. Howell's most important work was done in collaboration with G. Carl Huber and was a study of peripheral nerve regeneration, for which the two were awarded a prize by the American Physiological Society. Howell left for Harvard in 1892, but Warren Plimpton Lombard, having resigned from Clark University with most of the rest of the faculty, was glad to replace Howell in Ann Arbor. Lombard, who served until 1923, had a reputation as a dull teacher, but he thoroughly drilled students in the fundamentals of physiology applied to medicine. Lombard loved apparatus, and he was able to mount a complete laboratory course in physiology not only for medical, dental and homeopathic students but for those in the literary department as well. His most important piece of research was construction of the "Lombard balance" on which a man's loss of weight could be measured minute by minute, thereby permitting calculation of the metabolic rate.

Perhaps as the result of his collaboration with Howell, fresh from the heady atmosphere of Johns Hopkins, Howell's junior collaborator, G. Carl Huber, determined to obtain advanced training in microscopic anatomy. Huber spent an industrious year in Berlin as a student of Waldeyer, Benda and Ehrlich, and upon returning to Michigan he began a long career as a neuroanatomist, ending with collaboration with Elizabeth Crosby, and as an embryologist in which, among other things, he definitively determined the embryology of the kidney.

As the result of the Anatomy Act passed in 1867 and amended in 1875, there was an adequate supply of what was politely called "anatomical material," and a building devoted to gross anatomical dissection was completed in 1889. When Corydon La Ford died in 1894, Vaughan persuaded the Regents to elect, by a divided vote, J. Playfair McMurrich as Ford's successor. The opposition to McMurrich was based on the fact that he was a Johns Hopkins–trained biologist without an M.D. degree. In both teaching and research McMurrich quickly demonstrated a detailed mastery of human gross anatomy as well as of embryology. The Michigan tradition of long sessions in the dissection room and equally long sessions in the anatomy lecture room was solidified by McMurrich.

George Dock, Arthur Robertson Cushny, and Drugs

Victor Vaughan brought John Jacob Abel to Michigan as professor of materia medica and therapeutics the same year he brought George Dock. Abel did not accomplish much in Ann Arbor, partly for lack of equipment and partly because he was away much of the time. When Abel left for Johns Hopkins in 1893, Vaughan replaced him with Arthur Robertson Cushny, who, like Abel, had been a pupil of Oswald Schmiedeberg. Cushny remained in Ann Arbor five times as long as Abel, and he was more than five times as productive as a pharmacologist. While he was in Ann Arbor, Cushny defined the action of digitalis on the mammalian heart, demonstrated the osmotic nature of saline catharsis and proved the differential reabsorption of urea and salts by the renal tubules.[4] Cushny taught a laboratory course in pharmacology, and he wrote *A Textbook of Pharmacology and Therapeutics* that remained the standard for thirty years.[5] Cushny and Dock were good friends, and they often took long bicycle trips together.

Dock expected his students to consult Cushny's textbook if they did not already know its contents. Cushny had said in the introduction that his object in writing the book was "to show how far the clinical effects of remedies may be explained by their action on the normal body, and how far these in turn may be correlated with physiological phenomena. It necessarily follows that the subject is treated from the experimental standpoint, and that the results of the laboratory investigator are made the basis of almost every statement."[6] This contrasts sharply with Dock's attitude, for Dock's use of drugs was based on clinical experience rather than on experimental evidence. Dock's list of twenty drugs, a list he gave to each class, contained iron, arsenic, mercury, bismuth, lead and zinc. He once demonstrated a patient with argyria to warn students against the use of silver nitrate, but he also recommended silver nitrate as a styptic in a case of gastric hemorrhage. Dock regularly prescribed strychnine as a cardiac stimulant, and he used large doses. He once told the class that a timid pharmacist might refuse to fill his prescriptions. Dock eventually became defensive about strychnine, but he continued to use it as long as he was in Michigan. On the other hand, Dock scorned indiscriminate use of quinine for any fever, and he would not use an antipyretic because it obscured the natural course of a disease.

Dock's students were taught pharmacy in their early years in medical school, and they were expected to recognize preparations casually mentioned by Dock: Blaud's pills, Dover's powder, Huxham's tincture and Basham's mixture. If students did not recall them offhand, they could look up their composition in *The Dispensary of the United States of America* that had been edited by H. C. Wood, Dock's teacher at Pennsylvania.[7]

George Dock's Colleagues: The Clinicians

Dock's most important colleagues in the minor clinical specialties were Roy Bishop Canfield, William F. Breakey and William J. Herdman. Canfield was a German-trained otolaryngologist whose skill and judgment Dock respected. Breakey was a Civil War veteran and a self-trained syphilologist and dermatologist. Dock agreed with Breakey that syphilis should not be treated until secondary symptoms appear. Herdman was an enthusiastic practitioner of electrotherapeutics, and because he had much of the necessary apparatus to hand when Röntgen's discovery became generally known in 1896, he could begin X-ray diagnosis and treatment at Michigan. The X-ray plates Dock showed the students were made by a technician trained by Herdman. Herdman's most important accomplishment was to persuade Michigan's Joint Board of Asylums for the Insane to build and support a psychopathic hospital next to the University Hospital for the purpose of using the skills of the Michigan faculty in research on prevention and treatment of mental illnesses. On February 13, 1906, Dock told the students:

> Ladies and gentlemen, the first thing I want to talk about is with reference to certain work we now have the opportunity of doing in the psychopathic hospital, work that I consider of very great value to the class and a very useful opportunity. This work is required, and at the same time it is not our object to make it difficult for anybody. We can make in the psychopathic hospital all the S[tatus]. P[raesens]'s. You may think that is not much of a thing to do. You

think they have nothing else the matter with them except some difficulty which is in the cortex. That is far from being the case. Almost all have organic disease outside the brain. A large proportion have visceral disease in various parts of the body. It might be more instructive if that were not so, because nothing is better for a medical student now and then to go carefully and systematically over the normal body; it gives practice of considerable benefit when he comes to the pathological body. So we will have this work done by sending students to the patients and have it done as far as possible in alphabetical order. The rush consists in this: they brought down thirty-five patients at once, and it will take some time to get those first patients rounded up. After that they will come at the rate of one or two a week. Let me give you one more tip. Don't bother about the patient's psychical condition. They will do all sorts of things to confuse you. Many of them are somewhat fascinating people to talk to; but try to get along as much as possible without being too abrupt with them yet not being carried away by them. Try to keep them in the most amiable frame of mind you can, but don't wander off into family histories, or their views on medicine, theology, philosophy, etc.

Ten days later the students had not handed in the S.P.'s. A student said the patients are too excited, "they won't let us take them." Dock replied: "Well, I think it would be a good thing to go over again; maybe they have got them pacified by this time."

Dock's major clinical colleagues were Charles B. Nancrede in surgery and Reuben Peterson in obstetrics and gynecology.

Nancrede had graduated from the University of Pennsylvania's medical school in 1869, and he had appointments at the Jefferson Hospital, the Episcopal Hospital, the Crippled Children's Hospital and Pennsylvania's Eye and Ear Institute. Despite this multiplicity of appointments, Nancrede had only a small practice and no professorial appointment. This was because of his rough character. Everyone who knew him emphasized the difficulty of getting along with him. Consequently, he had plenty of spare time to teach anatomy at Pennsylvania, where George Dock was one of his students.

Nancrede was conservative in attitude. He would, for example, do no exploratory laparotomy, and he would do no palliative operation unless he were sure it would do the patient good. Nevertheless, along with W. W. Keen, he was among the first in Philadelphia to adopt antiseptic and then aseptic practice. He identified by electrical stimulation and then excised an epileptic focus long before that became a common operation. He is said to have been the first to perform an appendectomy in Philadelphia, and when he was in Ann Arbor he was equally adventurous in beginning biliary surgery. Because he needed the salary to support his wife and children, he was glad to accept Victor Vaughan's offer of the professorship of surgery at Michigan in 1889. Nancrede's Michigan colleagues did not like him, but they respected him. Dock's *Clinical Notes* show that Dock and Nancrede frequently consulted on the advisability of surgical intervention, and they record that Nancrede stayed in the hospital all night to perform an emergency repair of the perforated intestine of a patient with typhoid fever.

Reuben Peterson, the professor of obstetrics and gynecology, had, like Dock, a national reputation, and he was president of the American Gynecological Society and a founding member of the American College of Surgeons. Peterson and Dock got along well, and they were allies in frustrating Victor Vaughan's attempts to move the clinical years to Detroit. Because most deliveries were at home and because civic authorities refused to pay for hospitalization of pregnant unmarried girls, Peterson practiced little obstetrics in the University Hospital, but he was a busy gynecological surgeon. He performed hundreds of ventral suspensions of the retrodisplaced uterus as well as the whole range of radical pelvic surgery. Patients were frequently referred between the medical and gynecological clinics. Peterson believed the abdominal incision should be large enough to permit palpation of the gallbladder, and at least once Dock attempted to do so while Peterson operated.

George Dock's Colleagues: Aldred Scott Warthin

When Dock arrived in Ann Arbor, Michigan's professor of pathology was Heneage Gibbes, an Englishman who had accompanied Emanuel Klein to India to investigate the cholera epidemic and who did not believe that Koch's "comma bacillus" caused cholera. He did not believe the tubercle bacillus causes tuberculosis. There was a prolonged controversy between Gibbes and Vaughan, culminating in a vote by the Board of Regents in 1895 that the chairs of pathology and medicine be combined, with Dock as the occupant. Gibbes was thereby unseated.

Dock, who had been trained as a pathologist by Osler, Virchow and Paltauf and who had been professor of pathology at the University of Texas in Galveston in 1889–1891, was competent to fill the additional chair, but fortunately he had Aldred Scott Warthin to assume much of the burden. Warthin began as Dock's assistant in medicine in 1891, but soon thereafter he spent three successive summers in Germany and Austria studying pathology under Ziegler, Paltauf, Kolisko and other masters. Warthin at once took responsibility for autopsies and surgical pathology, and he began a laboratory course that for thirty-five years was notorious for its rigor. Warthin took over the lectures in pathology from Dock in 1898, and in 1903, on one of his trips to Germany, Warthin saw Dürer's *Ritter, Tod und Teufel* in a shop window; he bought it as the first of a collection that grew to 685 etchings, drawings and prints depicting Death. In 1931 he published a handsome volume, *The Physician of the Dance of Death*, based on his collection. He intended to present the first copy to Dock, inscribing it in a shaky hand:

> George Dock, from Aldred Scott Warthin, In Memory of the good times we had together in the 1890's

but Death danced off with him.

George Dock and the Medical Library

Each Michigan professor had been allowed $200 a year for books, but in the 1880s Victor Vaughan persuaded them to consolidate the funds in his hands as a regular appropriation for the medical library. By 1892 the library contained sixty-one medical periodicals, but only one, *Archiv für Anatomie und Physiologie*, was complete. There were also textbooks, many of them out of date.

Dock encouraged medical students to improve their education by systematic reading, including foreign journals in German, French and Italian. He thought that they should read medical classics and that, when they were in practice, they should combine with other doctors in the town to form a medical library. Vaughan was glad to make Dock chairman of the library committee in 1892. Dock worked quickly, and by 1895 he had completed from volume one all journals already taken. When he instituted new subscriptions, he bought full sets of back numbers. The result was that by 1905 the library contained 13,455 bound volumes and 266 journals of which 89 were complete. Warthin, who succeeded Dock as chairman, was proud that, although the medical library was part of a relatively young state university and that it had no endowment, it was the equal of medical libraries of some great eastern universities.

The University Hospital

None of the original medical faculty had any hospital training, and there was no community hospital in Ann Arbor until 1910. In 1856 and again in 1857, students were offered clinical instruction during the summer in a Detroit hospital, but few took advantage of the opportunity. Michigan graduates who wanted hospital experience went to New York or Philadelphia rather than to Detroit. The university converted one of the houses built for professors into a home where patients could stay until they were demonstrated in the medical building. As Victor Vaughan said: "There were no wards and no operating or dressing rooms, no place where students could receive bedside instruction." In 1878 the university built on campus a much larger pavilion hospital containing an operating theater. Its presence among other university buildings may be the reason President Angell insisted that the new University Hospital, begun in 1891, be as far away from the central campus as possible.

When George Dock arrived in Ann Arbor, the university was building two identical hospitals on Catherine Street, nearly half a mile from the central campus. One was for the regular medical school, and one was

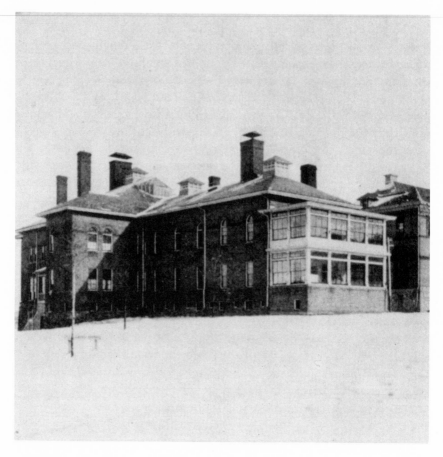

FIGURE 2. The University Hospital in the winter of 1902–1903. The building at the far right is the East Wing, used by surgery and the surgical specialties. The building in the middle is the Palmer Ward, used by pediatrics and other specialties. The building on the left is the West Wing, used by internal medicine and the medical specialties. The buildings were connected by a wooden corridor hidden by the Palmer Ward.

for the homeopathic school forced on the university by the legislature in 1875. The hospitals were being paid for by $50,000 appropriated by the legislature and by $25,000 voted by Ann Arbor citizens. The one to the east, used by the regular faculty including Dock, had an open ward of seventy-two beds, five obstetrical beds and twelve single rooms for very sick patients. The hospital had been designed by an architectural firm with little experience in hospital construction, and it had no classrooms and no laboratories of any kind. Students were taught and patients were demonstrated and operated upon in a small pit from which rose a semicircular array of uncomfortable wooden benches.

In 1901 the homeopathic department acquired a hospital of its own nearer the central campus, and internal medicine, together with neurology, dermatology and obstetrics, moved into the vacant space in what was thereafter called the West Wing of the University Hospital. The East Wing was left to surgery and surgical specialties. The two wings were connected by a long wooden corridor. In 1903 the Palmer Ward, intended for pediatrics and paid for by Alonzo B. Palmer's widow, was built between the two wings. Consequently, at the end of the period covered by the *Clinical Notes* Dock's service controlled about 114 beds in the wards and 20 beds in single rooms.[8]

After the spring vacation in 1908, Dock told the students:

> I must add that a curious chance in the hospital service shows itself. Not very long ago [to 1897] this hospital was only a college term hospital, only open during the college year, that is the professors came only on the clinic days, and the rest of the time kept as far away as possible, and so vacation was always a sort of time off; people did not come down and the internes died of ennui; but because patients discovered that there were not so many workers around and it was rather an easier time for them, it has happened for a number of years that vacations have been fuller than other times.

When Dock left Michigan in 1908, his colleagues Reuben Peterson said that Dock neglected his private practice in order to be in the hospital at all times.

In theory only indigent patients were admitted to the University Hospital, and their charges were borne by the county of residence or by the state of Michigan. All patients were used for teaching. Some patients who could afford to pay were admitted for one or another reason, and Dock sometimes admitted his own private patients so that they could be seen by the students. Consequently, there were occasional uproars in medical circles over admission of patients who could afford to pay for medical services. The university Regents received memorials and deputations in protest, and newspapers asserted that after "free medicine" the university would provide "free law." One regent from the Northern Peninsula, however, demanded to be taken care of in the University Hospital, and Dock, to discourage the practice, had senior medical students practice gastric lavage on him twice a day. The regent was pleased by the attention he received.

Eventually, admission was restricted to

1. Those whose admission is provided by special statutes,
2. Emergency cases,
3. All students in attendance at the university,
4. All persons bringing letters recommending their admission from their regular medical attendant, and
5. All persons applying for admission and not coming under the classes mentioned above who make an affidavit that he or she is financially unable to pay the usual minimum fees of the profession for treatment required.

George Dock's Students

Student's attending Dock's clinical demonstrations were in the fourth year of a four-year medical course. In order to be admitted to Michigan's medical school, students had to be matriculants in the literary department of the university or graduates of the classical course in high schools approved by the university. All must have satisfied requirements rigidly specified and occupying at least two college years. These included courses in English, mathematics through plane geometry, physics, botany, zoology, history and Latin. Some students had graduated from college.

Clinical work began in the students' third year and occupied all of the fourth year. Dock and his chief assistant gave lectures on internal medicine in the third year, and one day a week one of them conducted a diagnostic clinic similar to that given in the fourth year but more elementary in nature. Dock's senior assistant also taught a third-year course in the elements of physical diagnosis, and at least once a patient shown in the fourth-year clinic was black and blue for having been percussed by the third-year class.

Between 1899 and 1908 there were 67 to 104 students in a forth-year class. Eight to seventeen of them were women, and the *Clinical Notes* show that Dock treated the women exactly like the men. The only difference was that, whereas Dock usually addressed a man by his last name, he called a woman Miss or Mrs. So-and-so. However, there was no false gallantry in his address to the women, and he never patronized them as he made them palpate, percuss or auscultate a patient. In turn, there is no evidence of false modesty on the part of the women.

Students in both the third and fourth years were expected to consult Osler's *Principles and Practice of Medicine* and some of the other standard textbooks of the day. Dock said: " It is better to study Osler carefully than to buy a number of other books. However, students might consult one or another of the 'Systems' of medicine in the library." Once he recommended the novels of S. Weir Mitchell.

Dock had a substantial and, for the time, well equipped laboratory for clinical chemistry, and it was used by his assistants, the interns, and the fourth-year students living in the hospital and acting as interns. It could also be used by a student doing a special study, such as following sugar excretion by a diabetic patient. However, Dock bitterly regretted that there was no clinical chemistry laboratory that could be used by all students. When a student was working up a patient, Dock said that

the laboratory part of the examination, unfortunately, you will have to get from others; the condition of the urine and the blood you will have to get from the records in the laboratories. In the ideal condition every student ought to work them out for himself, but there are two things that prevent that, not only in this hospital, but in others. First, there isn't enough time; in the next place, there isn't room enough or apparatus enough to do it.

The Work of the Year

Dock began each year with a long description of the year's work. Once he said: "We are here to study medicine not only out of books but out of actual experience with patients. The method we pursue here is almost entirely what might be called catachistic, using the student as a victim and trying to work out not only all that we can about the patient but also what we can about the method and knowledge of the student."

The class was divided into sections of five or six students each, and a section met Dock in the morning on the wards four days a week for two weeks. A patient was assigned to each student in order, and a student was responsible for his patient until the patient was discharged. The student was to see the patient in his home if necessary; the student was to know what happened to his patient in other clinics; and he was to be present if the patient were operated upon. The student was to

[g]et into the habit, whenever he was called to see a sick person, of seeing him as promptly as possible and doing the work of investigation at once. The patient may change materially in a short time, he may die or leave and you would lose your work. What we will do now, will be for you in the first place, to take your patient's history. In the second place, to work out fully the physical examination. Make daily visits to the patients and go over the changes you found before, and to go over the history again in the light of which you have been studying; to make a diagnosis, and to give your reasons for the diagnosis and to make out a line of treatment, in other words to get everything you can out of the patient.

Dock repeatedly emphasized the primary importance of examining the patient. For example, when Dock questioned a student about a patient demonstrated three days before, he asked:

What do you think has been going on in your patient since you saw him before?

STUDENT: I have examined the records and have seen no development.

DOCK: Did you examine him in the ward? Don't you think that would have been the better place? In the first place, in the laboratory you have only second-hand information, so that you are leaning on some other man and the other man may be a cripple. You can learn a good deal more by seeing your patient for two minutes than by turning over the leaves of a record.

Sometimes a student had trouble finding a patient.

DOCK: The patient came in on the 15th, that was three days ago, and you were assigned when?

STUDENT: Yesterday at one o'clock.

DOCK: And you went to find him and the nurse said he was not in, and that shows that those most apparently infallible will be mistaken because he was in bed then. (To patient): Weren't you?

PATIENT: I haven't been out of the hall.

DOCK: So what I would like to emphasize from this experience is that when you are assigned, believe first, the assignment is right, in other words, that if assigned, the patient is around somewhere, and then be sure you have his name right, and when told that no such patient is around, remark that probably there is a mistake somewhere; necessarily you do that in a circumspect manner, but still you can do it in some way that the odium will come on somebody else besides yourself.

Histories were to be finished within twenty-four hours, and the results of the complete workup were to be handed in as soon as possible. To encourage good work Dock exempted those handing in the best reports from the final examination in June.

Dock knew his students had only eight or nine months of clinical experience before going into practice. He told them:

In Germany men have to work five semesters in clinics of various kinds in internal medicine before they can pass an examination; and after that a year in a hospital before they can get a degree, twelve semesters altogether, but seven semesters working wholly with sick people. Here where at the most you have two years, in some schools only one year, you can easily see that it requires all the superiority of the Anglo Saxon, especially as developed in the middle west of the United States, to accomplish the work in one year that others strive to accomplish in three and a half. . . . You come to see a patient with ascites. You realize you don't know much about tuberculosis of the peritoneum, have forgotten everything you ever knew about cirrhosis of the liver, and don't know ascites of nephritis, heart disease and so on. Don't lose your head, but work up the things you can, then hasten home to your text books and don't skip over them but carefully dig out what they say about the disease. If you know how to study and investigate a case, and if you have access to a fair textbook, you will be able to make yourself at home on practically any case that comes before you in practice. . . . Not long ago I was in the office of one of the most celebrated physicians in the country, and noticed a large number of 6 oz. bottles. On asking what they were for, he said, "When I don't know what is the matter with a patient I give him one of those and tell him to come back the next day with his urine. Then I have time to look up what is the matter with him."

Dock also knew students had other things to do. Once when a student said he had been too busy to see his patient, Dock questioned him sympathetically about what he had to do elsewhere. The student and six surgical patients to care for. Dock told the students: "If you are too busy, tell Dr. Arneill. Do not take [a case] at all unless you can do it carefully. There is nothing more disastrous to mental discipline and accuracy than to take a case about which you haven't time to think carefully and accurately." But another time he told a student he was a slave; slaves always have time.

At the Tuesday and Friday clinics students in the current section were expected to be in the pit of the theater with Dock to examine the patient and to answer questions. Patients drawn from the wards had already been examined by a student, usually not one in the current section. The student responsible for the patient was expected to be ready to answer questions as well, and Dock frequently called on other students to come down to examine the patient in the pit. As for the rest of the students: "They sit on their tubera ischia and hear the wisdom and mistakes of their colleagues." They should, however, learn from the patient's voice, judge his exact age, height, and weight, anticipate questions and answers and cultivate diagnosis by inspection.

Students did learn something under Dock, and toward the end of the year they characteristically showed more knowledge and self-confidence than they had earlier. Once a woman student skeptically questioned by Dock replied flatly: "I know I am right."

How to Behave

At the first clinic Dock told the students:

Most of you are now being brought for the first time in communication with sick people, and have to do with people who throw themselves upon the mercies of doctors and medical students. In the first place, remember that all patients that come here, come here for your benefit. They come to this hospital partly because it has a reputation as a hospital, but also because they know they will be used as teaching material. They know they will be handled by cold hands, and sometimes by septic hands. They come here because they think that good will be done them and that it will out balance any harm that will be done. They look upon you as a doctor, and immediately the amount of faith these people put in you, let alone a doctor, is almost incredible. . . . Try to remember even, if the humanitarian part is not strong, the more carefully they are treated, the more likely are you to have useful material in this hospital. Aside from that, these patients, although they may seem nothing at all to you, are, after all, human, as your fathers and mothers or sisters are human, and should be treated as considerately as they, and as you would wish them treated if they were similarly placed.

But, Dock said:

they look upon you as young and tender. The patient uses these qualities to "work you," as the ordinary expression is. They will come to you in this way, they will say, what does the doctor think of my case? Tell him you do not know. An infinite amount of harm has been done in just these ways, the unwise imparting of information that is not yours to the patient. Do not say, Your prognosis is bad, and you will not get well. Try to cultivate reticence. For medical students to talk among themselves I regard as harmless. Don't talk outside the hospital, at the boarding house table "I have a peach of a cancer." Even in the hospital it is possible for one to be rather reckless in the use of his tongue. One of the greatest temptations with me is to refrain from speaking of a patient as an "interesting case." I always try to use the word instructive. . . . The gossipy doctor is an abomination, and let me warn you, let me strongly urge you to guard against even the semblance of such a course.

Patients

There is no way of telling how the patients Dock demonstrated represented the patient population on the wards, for the hospital records of the period have been destroyed. Dock apparently chose patients to illustrate major medical problems. There were always typhoid fever cases and patients in all stages of tuberculosis. Sometimes Dock would show three thyroid patients at once. However, a substantial number of outpatients who had never been seen before wandered into the clinic, and Dock used them as examples of office practice. Then as epidemics occurred there were patients with scarlet fever, smallpox or diphtheria.

Dock and his colleagues on the faculty were always sensitive to the criticism that, because Ann Arbor had a population of only twenty thousand, their clinical material must be small. He thought that the University Hospital with more than two hundred beds was large enough, for the beds were always full and all patients were used for teaching. He said:

> There are hospitals much larger than this where the comparison is out of the question, the General Hospital in Vienna with 3,000 beds, the University Hospital of the Medical School in Berlin with 1,600 beds, and they are to build a Hospital costing $4,000,000 and everything else in proportion; and yet even in those very large hospitals one can live for a year on the wards without seeing examples of various diseases that might be encountered in practice.

Dock had helped frustrate Dean Vaughan's repeated attempts to move the clinical years to Detroit, and after one such episode he said:

> For example, students are sometimes heard suggesting that if we were in some city not more than four or five thousand miles away

we should have such and such opportunities; yet we know we have more cases of fever, diseases of the heart, important diseases of the lungs and blood than occur in a great many larger hospitals. For example, we have been able to see every year some of the acute diseases, smallpox, measles, scarlet fever, diphtheria, and even plague. We don't talk about that so much. . . . The point is, What is really available for actual handling by medical students? and in that respect we are peculiarly fortunate right here. While we haven't all we would like to have, yet what we have we are able to utilize fairly thoroughly.

Children were the one group missing, and students asked for special work in pediatrics. Dock told them:

Children's diseases don't differ from those of grown people. If you know internal medicine and surgery, physiology and pathology of adults you know all these diseases in children, but the matter of investigating children's diseases is quite different from that of adults, especially before the age of talking. So that in the study of the practical diagnosis of children, we always find a great deal of difficulty in investigating. You can't learn how to diagnose children's diseases out of books any more than you can learn to skate out of a book.

Students had asked for lectures and a quiz course in pediatrics, and despite Dock's opinion about learning from books, he said:

If you can't get this hour you can still do something in the next few months by putting in a few minutes or a couple of hours now and then reading. If you want to get a book that is to children's diseases about the same as Osler to internal medicine, then I would advise you to get Holt's "Diseases of Children." It is not so much the description of diseases you want; but the introductory chapters concerning the methods of examining children and you can get that much more quickly by reading than from the best lectures anybody could give. You will be able to read on the nutrition of the child, which is very important. The first baby you will be called upon to see or bring into the world will have, probably, to be artificially fed, and, unless you know how this is done, you will begin as a slovenly practitioner and continue the bringing up of atrophic babies. Then another important thing is convulsions. You can read about them quite as well as you can hear the most eloquent lecturer talk about them. I always speak about this time of year [February] of the importance of studying children's diseases particularly because you have to know about them. Children are more liable to be your first patients than grown people. People will trust children to the young doctor when they won't trust themselves.

Later in 1904 Dock told the students that "the Faculty listened with gracious ears to your petition, and left the matter in my hands." An hour was made available for pediatrics, and Dock used it to quiz on Holt's textbook. He continued to demonstrate pediatric patients now and then.

Examinations

Dock sometimes reviewed midterm examinations. Once, after discussing medical mistakes some students made, he said:

I think it can be said that there are three or four people who worked out a process commonly known as bluffing. They wrote very nice papers if you did not think what they were writing. They were filled with lore and fine expression; that goes well with me because I am an easy mark, but if any of you try that on certain state boards you will find yourself among the missing. I still find reason for criticising certain points with reference to such matters as English and spelling. I never mark a man down because of his spelling and English, no matter how bad they are. But medicine is more and more a learned profession, and men in it are supposed to have a preliminary education, and one of the ear marks is a fairly accurate use of English and fairly accurate method of spelling. Of course I know very well that people who can spell very well in the haste of an examination will make a lot of mistakes, for example, get an e and a wrong in a word like separate. But there are certain things, for example, when a man doesn't know how to write crescentic, but calls it "crescentric", and persistently misspells disease, spelling it with two s's together, it is somewhat different from spelling college and knowledge wrong. What a man who is obliged to deal in new scientific literature has to do is to use his eyes so carefully that he sees the words correctly. So, for example, when a man spells sternum "stur", it doesn't look as if that man was competent to pass a scientific opinion on the sternum. There are, of course, certain names very difficult to spell properly; but when a man spells, for example, a word like Koplik, "lick" or "lig", I think it is doubtful whether he will know the spots. If a man persistently speaks of a "tubercule", how do I know he can tell a tubercle when he sees it? Let me urge you to pay attention to these little points and in future papers try to avoid them.

EXAMINING
THE PATIENT

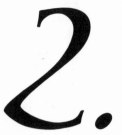

AT THE BEGINNING OF EACH YEAR
Dock gave detailed instructions in history taking, and throughout the
year he had many opportunities to criticize histories. He gave much
sketchier directions on how to do a physical examination at that time,
for students were relentlessly drilled on the subject later.

Eliciting the History

Dock said that in taking a history it is better to follow a tried and true
method, just as a bricklayer learns from skilled workmen. Nevertheless,
the process is not stereotyped. Any clerk, he said, might take a history if
he had a scheme and got answers "yes and no," but such a history would
be very different from that taken by an expert who knew how to put
things together and in what order to bring out points.

> The art of history taking consists; in drawing out a point the pa-
> tient doesn't know, and the ability to do that depends upon a
> knowledge of the disease. The physician impresses the patient that
> he knows what he is doing when he asks leading questions. . . . In
> the first place, the patient very often has the idea that it is unneces-
> sary for you to do the work and look on you as being personally re-
> sponsible for bothering them. It is important, then, to explain to
> the patient that you are not doing this for fun—and I dare say that
> statement would be perfectly true—and not doing it out of idle cu-
> riosity, but doing it really for the patient's good. The patients don't
> know that you are beginners; they think most of you are doctors;
> of course they call you students and talk about your experiment-

26

ing, but really in their hearts they think you are all right. . . . We have found it useful to follow a plan followed in most teaching hospitals and for the convenience of students I have put it in a little book called "Outlines of Case-taking" that can be found in the book stores.[1] [The plan] consists in the first place in taking the patient's name, age, married condition, position, etc. Following this, we make a statement that is used now in a good many hospitals, although it is not described in all the text books and not given in all schemes printed in books for case-taking. This consists in taking the patient's chief complaint first.

Most patients, Dock said, will tell you at once why they came.

DOCK: For example, let us ask this patient what she complains of. (To patient): What do you complain of?

PATIENT: Of a bad feeling in my left side.

DOCK (TO STUDENTS): That is very good. The patient says she complains of a pain or bad feeling in her left side, and you would naturally go on and find out exactly where it is in the left side. But in many cases the answer is entirely different; the patient will say with a look of surprise, not unmixed with scorn, that is what she came to find out. She thinks you are asking what disease she has. It is important to say to a patient, and in a kind hearted way, that what you want is the symptoms and not the name of the disease.

At a later clinic a student began:

The Doctor said . . .

DOCK: Let me call attention to one thing. I notice in a good many histories too much attention paid to what the Doctor said. It is well not to do this for two reasons. In the first place, any sort of history you get second hand is likely to be misleading; second, it is a good thing to leave that part of the history out. Try to get the patient to describe his symptoms at that time, but when he tries to explain what the doctor thought he had you get a wrong impression. The doctor may not have told him what he thought about it. He is just as likely to give him a partial answer. Then it opens the ground for too much discussion of the other doctor's treatment. The patient's description may be altogether wrong and the doctor may hear some remarks which you passed which may have been equally wrong. Finally, it is of no value.

Dock said the family history must be complete according to the nature of the disease:

In many schemes the family history comes later, but the general tendency has been to have the family history come immediately after the first statement and has this advantage, if you clear up the family history you are through with it and have it off your hands. The family history is useful in this way, it gives a good chance to study the psychological condition of sick people. You learn how they talk about sick people, how intelligent they are, and have a chance of stimulating your own minds and will learn to think more quickly on all those things otherwise. In getting the family history you take it in the natural order, beginning with the father and mother, then usually the grandparents and immediate collateral relatives, that is uncles and aunts. It is enough as a usual thing not to go farther back, although there may be reasons for doing so. For example, if the patient is a congenital bleeder then we can't go too far back, we should go as far as memory can carry him or even find out by correspondence.

The patient's personal history comes next, "the history of the physiological condition and pathological conditions as far back as he can remember. Some know much, some little, and it is usually to the patient's credit that he does not know about it. The patient who knows a great deal usually causes a good deal of trouble." As to a patient's occupation, Dock observed that one who was a jeweler may not get any outdoor exercise. When a student said that nothing in a patient's occupation throws any light on his disease, Dock responded that it is necessary to ask more closely. Knowing that the patient is a hotel keeper means he is exposed to alcoholic drinks. When questioned, the patient said he often took liquor and sometimes a great deal of it. Another saloon keeper swore he was a teetotaler.

As for "habits," Dock continued:

In acute disease it makes little difference unless his habits have been of an unusually bad kind. In a case of typhoid fever if the patient is a chronic drinker it makes a difference, but if he takes a glass of beer now and then or smokes a cigarette occasionally it is of trifling moment. But if it is a case of neurosis or cardiac or gastric disease that may be influenced by such things, then we have to investigate all the habits of eating and drinking and the use of intoxicants of all kinds. In many cases it is unnecessary to investigate the sexual life and in many cases it is absolutely necessary, and when we have to get it the thing to do is to go at it in such a way as to get it. So it is often a waste of time to ask whether the patient has this or that specific disease; he doesn't know the names, but if you ask in the vernacular you will find that he is nearly always instructed and if he isn't then you will have to ask about symptoms, trying in all cases to get perfectly clear and unmistakable answers. In the case of women it is not always well to ask direct questions, for the reason that women don't always know; so we try to find out indirectly by asking about menstrual history, uterine diseases, etc.

Dock had many opportunities to criticize histories, for most patient presentations began with the student reading the history. Once Dock said:

We are not talking about the patient now; we are having an inquest on the history.

STUDENT: I think it is all right.

DOCK: I think that is a safe verdict to make. The history is a good history. At the same time this is not a love feast, but a place for instruction, so if there is anything at all you think could be improved in the history let us hear about it. Just as when Tolstoi reads Shakespeare he thinks he could improve it a little. The only thing I could suggest is that we try to avoid figurative or poetic expressions. We don't say "suffered" or was "afflicted." They belong on a man's epitaph and have no place in a history than they would have in a bank balance sheet. So while I would not like to discourage any ardent soul from throwing all the poetry he can into this life of ours, yet it would be well to leave it off the history.

At another time there was a flagrant example:

Here is the sort of history I feel compelled to criticize. "Has gone out with the boys and imbibed the amber colored liquids, etc." That would be all right at a minstrel show, but you would not want to have a doctor come into your office and look over your card catalogue and see a note of that kind.

A student should cut short his questions if they tire the patient, but

It will be very much better to do too much than too little. The time in actual practice is too short for the sort of drill we are getting here, but if you take extensive histories it is easy to get into the habit of sorting the essential things later, and form judgment that makes this possible.

The Physical Examination

Dock gave directions for making a physical examination:

In working the present condition of your patient you will have to do the best you can with the limited room we have here. Very often you will have to work in the wards, you will have to work in the noise, probably the best you can do is put a screen around the patient. Go over your patient thoroughly. First try to find out from the history what you are likely to find in the patient's body. Then go over the organs that are likely to be affected, and then over those that are not likely to be affected. In doing this we usually follow an anatomical order, but very often we vary these according to the nature of the disease so that if a patient's symptoms are limited to the diseases of the chest such as consumption, we usually begin with the respiratory tract.

Inspection

DOCK: First, the eyes.

STUDENT: I don't see anything the matter with them.

DOCK: Your eyes, I mean, not hers.

The patient must be completely exposed, and sometimes Dock had trouble with that. When he asked three students their opinion of a fully-dressed outpatient and got three different answers, Dock said: "So here is a good example of how a person may be extremely emaciated and not show it with his clothes on. We can't draw any conclusions about a sick man without seeing him all over."

Dock complained about the hospital routine:

We all suffer here from the failure of patients to be properly clothed. Whether he belongs to the pajama wearing class or not he should be put into them because that garment is convenient for physical examination, and then slippers or socks, and then he should wear those things as long as he is in the hospital. It is easy to unbutton the pajamas and examine over the whole body; whereas by having a woolen undershirt and then by having a blue flannel shirt of the heaviest quality over it, it is extremely difficult to do anything for the patient, especially if he complains bitterly every time you touch him. I don't know that any hospital has reached the point now occupied by the smart set where women wear pajamas too, but the mother hubbard answers a similar purpose, that is, that it is a loose ill-fitting garment, so that you can easily make any examinations necessary over it.

Such dress has a social advantage.

In the first place, under such conditions, the patients are all alike. You all know how unpleasant it is when one patient, especially in the female ward, has a silk waist and another cheaper ones. All ought to be on the same footing in the sick room. In Germany we had no trouble at all.

When Dock's rule was broken, he said:

> Just why he has his night shirt on I am at a loss to understand. I suppose we ought to be thankful that he doesn't have his evening clothes on. (To nurse): It is a standing order to have shirts off on all occasions.

And at another time:

> I thought I said not to do that any more, let whoever put it on come take it off. It is as shocking as the figures you see in the Vatican Museum where they have put petticoats on the Madonnas. Never put those things on; if there is anything that isn't fit to be seen in a clinic, we don't bring it in.

The transcript records that of all the patients demonstrated in eight years, only three women patients wanted their faces covered when they were being examined before the class.

Dock was careful in examining a patient's skin. He asked of a patient referred from surgery:

> What do you think of his skin that you can see?
>
> STUDENT: It seems pigmented in both inguinal regions.
>
> DOCK: Part of that pigmentation looks like what? It looks like dirt. One of the unfortunate features about this place is the difficulty to bathe our patients because we haven't enough bath tubs. Every man who comes into the hospital unless he is obviously too sick to have a bath, that is, injured or wounded or otherwise very sick, ought to have a bath in hot water with green soap and it is usually a good thing to add kerosene to the soap.

Dock looked at the patient's expression as well.

> DOCK: Where is Larson? Larson you are too far away. Come down a little nearer the scene of action. What do you think about his face?
>
> STUDENT: It is rather serious.

DOCK: This isn't psychology. Miss Crozier?

STUDENT: There are lines around his mouth. It is a little more drawn than usual.

DOCK: The nasolabial fold is very marked. We don't pay as much attention to these things as we ought. They have more medical interest than psychological, and such a line as that is often associated with abdominal disease. For example, if you notice an old dyspeptic, he nearly always has lines down around his mouth. If he has disease in the thorax you find he has alterations in the middle of his face, about his nose; if he has obstruction or disease in the lungs he will often have moving alae nasi; if he has pain in the head he will show it in the upper part of his face. There will be wrinkles across his forehead or eyes. These are small but important things.

Dock told how to begin examining a patient with a cough:

I say to him "pull up your shirt" and he begins very slowly and as he does so he generally talks, and tells me more about his case. Naturally we cannot treat all people the same and we would not give the same sort of order to a sensitive woman that we would give to an ordinary man. In such cases you say to the patient something like this: You have symptoms that make it highly probable that you have something wrong with the organs in your chest, and I will have to examine the chest. You ask the patient if she wears corsets, if you cannot tell from her external appearance. And you can examine under the next thing she wears. Such a thing is nearly always distasteful to a woman and that brings up a more important point. The examination of the thorax in such a woman is much more disagreeable to her than to examine the abdomen. You come against a feeling of modesty that is quite natural, so that you have to get along without offending that feeling too much. So you begin by examining through the clothing. But you cannot examine the chest through a corset of any kind. They interfere with the lung and liver boundary and with the lower part of the thorax in the back. So that even there you have to insist quietly, as if it were a perfectly natural procedure, on those things being out of the way. Where you can be satisfied pretty well there are no lesions you can get the stethoscope down under the garment, and also percuss over the garment. But if there is an obscure lesion you will have to tell the patient you must examine directly over the chest. More mistakes are made by neglecting that practice in women perhaps than from ignorance of the subject.

Palpation

Dock told his students that if they knew how to do a good physical examination they could solve almost any medical problem. Many older physicians did not know how to do that, and when his students were out in practice old physicians would call on them to palpate, percuss, and auscultate. "Don't let them rattle you." Consequently, Dock drilled his students in technique.

Now suppose you go ahead and palpate him. There you are probably somewhat handicapped by your cold hands. The patient is in bad condition to palpate because he is shivering himself. A good way to do is to warm your hands on the patient by examining some other parts; for example, the thorax or heart. . . . You never creep with your fingers over the abdomen. There is nothing more disagreeable. The first thing you know, you get the patient's muscles contracting, and then you cannot do anything. . . . You hold your fingers too stiff. . . . Remember a man was given five fingers in order to be able to palpate with all of them. It was never supposed he would use only one.

When a student tried to feel the spleen, Dock said:

In order to feel the spleen one should know where it is. That saves time. We always feel the spleen standing on the right side. Anybody who goes away with an examination on the left side and says the spleen is negative, makes a very serious mistake. When you feel about the end of the 10th rib you feel something coming up against your fingers. Get the patient to take a deep breath, and then if the spleen is enlarged you feel it coming up against your

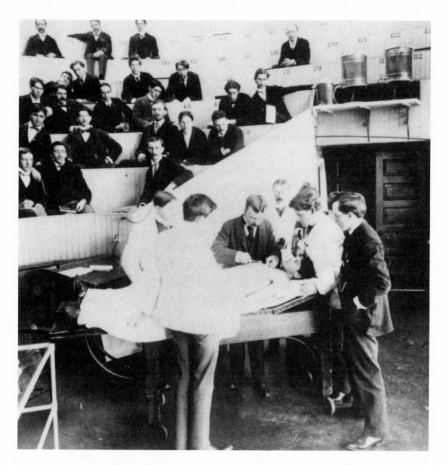

FIGURE 3. George Dock purportedly examining a patient in one of his diagnostic clinics. James Arneill is standing behind Dock's left shoulder, and the students in the section surround the patient. The patient, however, is wearing street shoes, and in view of Dock's insistence that patients be completely exposed, it is obvious that a medical student posed as the patient for the sake of the picture. Dock is using a hammer for percussion.

fingers rather abruptly. Sometimes you feel it just as the diaphragm goes back again. Suppose you palpate again and I will show you something. Get your finger right at the edge, then press your finger back and then up toward her head and then upward. Can't you feel the edge now? Now that is a very important little trick to use when you are feeling any organ that has an edge in the abdomen. If you press down you may not feel it, but if you put your finger under it and then push it ahead of you toward the skin you get down under it.

Sometimes a patient's abdomen was too distended to be palpated, and sometimes it was too rigid. In the latter case:

DOCK (to nurse): Now we want a large compress, nurse, right away, large enough to cover his abdomen and as hot as he can stand it. I can tell you a better way to wring that out if you have another towel. The way to do it is to take a kitchen fork and pull the towel out of the boiling water or turpentine or whatever you have; lay it on the other towel, and then let two people twist it. In that way you don't burn yourself at all, and yet the thing stays hot.

At another time Dock said the patient might be examined in a hot bath. "Immerse the patient in a bath of about 100 degrees, run it up to 110 degrees and in that way relax the abdominal wall, and we would be able to find things that we would not otherwise."

And an example of student competence:

STUDENT: He has a new growth of some kind, two or three of them. He has one on the right testicle, another at the internal abdominal ring, and this growth in the abdomen.

DOCK: Tell us more about the growth in his testicle.

STUDENT: It is very hard, has a peculiar feel.

DOCK: How much larger is the testicle than the other one?

STUDENT: Perhaps a quarter larger.

DOCK: Yes, and it is thicker and very hard, and the hardness occupying what part? . . . Another important thing is the character of the vas deferens. Is that altered or not? What do you think?

STUDENT: It is not enlarged.

Percussion

Dock had read Auenbrugger's *Inventum novum ex percussione thoracis humani ut signo abstrusos interni pectoris morbos detegendi,*[2] and when he taught percussion he said: "This is old Auenbrugger's percussion with all fingers although he probably percussed over a shirt with a glove on."

There used to be a tradition that a body had to strike three times. There are several objections to this. First, it is not necessary; when percussing small areas, you can run a great risk of getting your ear confused by what you have heard before, so I would strongly suggest that the habit of percussing only once when you are percussing something that is fairly well defined. Then there is a disadvantage in percussing short distances, for example, say the apex beat is here, then it is not very much displaced and the probabilities are that the upper border of the heart dulness is not very high up. Now there isn't very much space between the clavicles and this point, so if you make two or three long steps you are likely to strike the dulness without much loss of time. So you begin and percuss, for example, in this way you get the difference right away. Then that brings one to the next point, you have to percuss as lightly as possible to bring out the note. For example, that brings out the note, doesn't it? So there we get a change, somewhere down there and there. There is the border, isn't there? See! Isn't it easier?

During percussion the boundaries were often marked on the patient's body with a soft pencil. Once the student could not find the heart. Dock said,

When we put marks on him he looks like the image of a man with proper marks as seen in a mirror. We run across such a case here every year or two, and see them in other places, and it is interesting to see how they can be overlooked. For example, we had a patient whom Dr. Cowie saw first in his office and found a condition of this kind, telling the man about it, and the man told him he had passed an examination for life insurance and been treated for pleurisy, and none of the other doctors had ever spoken of it. When a patient complains of a pain in that part of his body it makes a great deal of difference whether he has his heart there or his lungs or his liver.

Auscultation

The patient was a university student with rheumatism. After percussion Dock asked:

Now what is the matter with his heart?

STUDENT: He has a loud blowing murmur which reflects the first sound at the apex.

DOCK: But what causes that?

STUDENT: It is caused by mitral regurgitation.

DOCK: Has he any other signs of mitral regurgitation?

STUDENT: The sound is conveyed out to the axilla.

DOCK: Well, what else? What else do you hear? Where is it loudest?

STUDENT: Just to the left of the sternum.

DOCK: What else is there?

STUDENT: Then there is a diastolic murmur in the right second intercostal space. There is a slight accentuation of the second pulmonic.

DOCK: Well, is there anything else in the aortic area?

STUDENT: There is also a murmur, a systolic murmur.

DOCK: Is it conducted anywhere? Did you hear it in the neck? Did you listen for it?

STUDENT: Not especially.

DOCK: Wouldn't it be a good thing to do? Suppose you come up and auscult this, More. What do you think?

STUDENT: I get a sound below the carotid.

DOCK: A sound or a murmur? By sound we mean a tone that isn't murmurish, a pure sound. Now is it further transmitted? Is it transmitted up in the neck? You want to be careful not to produce murmurs, for example, Mr. Work pressed too hard. By listening with very soft pressure over there you get a murmur, and then you can also hear it over the subclavian just as it comes out from under the carotid. Did you follow it there? That would be a good thing to do. Do you hear it?

STUDENT. It is faint.

DOCK: I know, but that is the point. If we only heard loud sounds we would not have to take the trouble to listen carefully. You can't expect your patients to go around with sirens on them.

Dock called on two more students to auscultate, and there are more pages of transcript before he summed up:

So he has a systolic murmur transmitted up toward the axilla; a double murmur in the aortic area, first transmitted to the great vessels and then backward; so that corresponds to a lesion in the aortic valves; impurity and stenosis and a certain amount of regurgitation. Then if the diagnosis is all right we ought to find something in his pulse. How about the vessels?

Autopsies

Some patients died in the University Hospital, and the ultimate examination occurred at autopsy. Dock said:

I need not point out that it is not discreditable to have such patients die. The common mind associates exactly the wrong standpoint with this; and this calls to mind what I read a short time ago. Some persons brought up a law in some state that all doctors were to report causes of death, and these and the number together. Statistics of that kind would not throw any discredit on any doctor from a doctor himself. The more cases a doctor has, the more deaths he will have; the more reputation, the more bad cases, and ergo, the more deaths. That is as easy as a proposition in Euclid, and if such statistics were kept up they would show whom the bad cases are going to, and other bad cases would go there.

The same applied to a hospital; the efficacy of a general hospital can always be expressed in the death rate. The better the reputation of a hospital, the higher the death rate.

On March 27, 1900, Dock told the class:

> We have had an unusual experience lately. Four patients died in 3 days and out of four deaths we had two autopsies. The fact that of the four patients who died within the last few days, only two have come to autopsy is a deplorable thing. The objection to making autopsies is purely sentimental. It prevails in this country largely because doctors do not make constant effort to make autopsies in practice.

Dock knew doctors who had no trouble getting autopsies because people had come to expect it. Dock remarked:

> People of Hibernian descent object to making autopsies. You sometimes find that Roman Catholics object to making autopsies. That is not because they are Roman Catholic, but have grown up in a country where this is objected to. I think I can speak on the subject, having lived in a Catholic hospital for a year, and have never had any trouble, because where people felt any objection at all, a word from the Priest or one of the nuns got their permission. In Austria, where everybody is Roman Catholic, and in Italy, the head center of Romanism, as you might say, nobody would think of declining to have an autopsy made any more than they would decline to have a doctor in the house if anybody was sick.

Autopsies at Michigan

When Dock arrived in Ann Arbor in 1891, Michigan's professor of pathology was Heneage Gibbes, who did not believe that tubercle bacilli cause consumption. Gibbes was dismissed by the university Regents in 1895 by the maneuver of combining the chair of pathology with that of internal medicine. Dock lectured on pathology from 1895 to 1898. In the meantime Aldred Scott Warthin, Dock's assistant, went to Germany and Austria in the summers to be trained as a pathologist. After 1895 Warthin did most of the work of teaching pathology in the laboratory and examining surgical specimens and performing autopsies. In 1903 Warthin was formally placed in charge of pathology.

Autopsy protocols have been preserved; they show that despite Dock's strictures very few autopsies were performed in his time at Michigan. The number ranges from a low of twelve in 1903–1904 to a high of thirty-three in 1904–1905. Those numbers include autopsies done out of term time and on patients dying on services other than internal medicine.

One reason for failure to obtain an autopsy was the family's promise that none would be done. When a young girl died of pneumonia following a mastoid operation, Dock was unable to get permission. He said: "The father was willing to have it made, but he was unfortunate in having been asked by the sick girl not to allow autopsy, and then her father being an honest man thought he ought to keep his promise. I have had lots of cases where people doubtless had had the same kind of Sunday School teacher I had, who thought a bad promise had better be broken than kept."

In 1901 a patient with a mass in his abdomen presented a particularly difficult problem. In a long differential diagnosis following an equally long physical examination, Dock could not decide whether the mass was primary or secondary and if secondary, of what? The proper course was to explore the patient, but the size of the growth and the exhaustion of the patient made the possibility of doing him any good remote. The patient died, but before death his family agreed there should be no autopsy. Nevertheless, an autopsy was performed; a tumor was found in the liver, but there was no disease of the stomach, pancreas, or gallbladder. No primary could be found for the reason Dock twice emphasized to the students: the autopsy was "hurried and incomplete." The records in the Department of Pathology contain no autopsy protocol, and the inference that the autopsy was done without permission is justified.

On a later occasion Dock told the class of a patient who had died of leukemia: "An autopsy was made—unfortunately it had to be very private." In this instance permission was given by the patient's husband. For some unknown reason the autopsy protocol is headed by the number XV, 159 I-XV, and the patient's name, but the protocol is otherwise totally blank.

CARDIOVASCULAR PROBLEMS

3.

EACH YEAR DOCK DEMONSTRATED
the thorough physical diagnosis of cardiovascular problems. Students must use their eyes and hands first and then their brains; an examination made without prejudice as to diagnosis should precede interpretation of findings.

Inspection

Once a student said the patient had a ruddy complexion. Dock convinced him that the patient's face was really livid and cyanotic and that his body was pale and yellow. The feet were edematous, and edema reached as far as the scrotum. Hands were cold, and the swollen feet were cold as ice.

DOCK: Lewis, what do you think?

STUDENT: It is due to poor circulation.

DOCK: "Poor circulation" as I have pointed out before is an extremely convenient word, but unless you know what you mean by it not a very good word to use among professionals. Poor circulation is the thing we tell the patient because he doesn't know what you mean by tension and back pressure and all those things.

Palpation: The Pulse

Palpation began with feeling the pulse. Is the radial artery straight or is it beaded? Dock said:

42

The way to tell is by putting the fingers on one of them and feeling the wall. You want to put three fingers on and you can tell by the way the fingers are on the artery whether it is reasonably straight or not. If the artery is crooked, the fingers will not be in a line. . . . It has a feel that we describe as being beaded. These beads are about 1/16 inch apart and so even that it gives the feel of the trachea of a small animal, so this has long been known as the goose trachea radial.

Blood pressure, or arterial tension, was estimated from the pulse:

DOCK: Suppose you feel his pulse, what about that? Is it large or small?

STUDENT: It is pretty fair sized, I think. I can't feel the vessel wall now.

DOCK: You can't feel it very well, but you call that fair sized? Well, now, feel your own. If his is fair sized then yours must be immense.

STUDENT: Do you mean the size of the wave?

DOCK: I mean the pulse itself, the whole sensation.

STUDENT: Well, it is weak.

DOCK: We haven't got to that yet. The question is whether it is large or small.

STUDENT: It is small.

DOCK: It is very small, isn't it? How about the sensation of speed in the waves, is it quick or slow?

STUDENT: I think it is rather quick.

DOCK: Now would you say that the tension is high or low? How do you tell? Is it hard or easy to compare?

STUDENT: I think it is about medium tension.

DOCK: What would you call medium tension? It seems small to me now and very low, and yet the tension taken this morning [October 25, 1904] was 140 mm. and that would be rather high. Now what else do you want to find out about the pulse?

STUDENT: The rate.

DOCK: Well, that is another more important point still. It does not feel dicrotic, does it? Suppose you palpate the heart.

STUDENT: Oh, the relation between the pulse and the heart.

DOCK: Yes, we know that one of the most certain guides to a loss of compensation is the disproportion between the apex beat and the pulse. Now here is a patient with a heaving apex beat. If he had compensation the pulse should be very strong.

STUDENT: The heart seems to be working very hard for the amount of pulse.

DOCK: That there is some insufficiency and we don't think there can be very much doubt about it.

Heart Rate and Rhythm

A patient's heart rate was often counted in the clinic. Patients with ex-ophthalmic goiter always had high rates, but sometimes Dock thought a moderate acceleration could be attributed to the patient's excitement at being shown. If each pulse wave were strong and clear, an accurate count could be made well above 180. Dock said that then one should feel the pulse, observe the watch at the same time, and count for only one-sixth of a minute. Experienced pulse-takers got into the habit of counting every other pulse. For a patient with arrhythmia, a nurse had once put the wrong heart rate in the chart because not all audible beats had been felt at the wrist.

Dock made many objective records of irregular pulse and pathologi-cal pulse forms with a sphygmograph, and he frequently showed the records to the students. He published records as well. Some taken in 1902 and published in 1905 are from patients with Stokes-Adams syn-drome.[1] Dock's colleague Arthur Cushny had studied the tracings and had diagnosed "diminished automatic excitability." This was before "Erlanger's beautiful and convincing experiments"[2] had shown the na-ture of partial and complete heart block. At another time Dock pub-lished a sphygmogram showing occasional extrasystoles followed by compensatory pauses, but he seems not to have recognized the reason for what he called " a very irregular rate."[3]

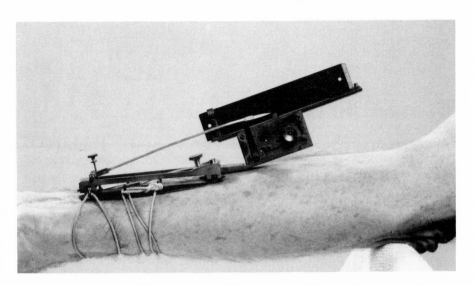

FIGURE 4. A sphygmograph from Michigan's Department of Physiology. The impulse from a foot resting on the radial artery is transmitted to the lever, whose point writes on a strip of smoked paper moved at a uniform rate by clockwork. Dock once showed a sphygmogram made in the Department of Physiology, and perhaps it was made with this instrument.

By November of 1907 Dock had obtained a polygraph, and while his assistant Dr. Van Zwaluwenburg demonstrated its use, Dock described its advantages over the "old-fashioned sphygmograph": It has two tambours, and it costs $120. It is so heavy that it doesn't take very delicate tracings. There is a Swiss instrument costing $50 that is a sphygmograph with one tambour and is easier to use. A polygraph with a continuous roll of paper will make tracings running one-half hour, but it is not on the market yet. Dock mentioned Mackenzie's book[4] and said:

The attachment we have on now is known as MacKenzie's polygraph because James Mackenzie living in the little town of M . . . . . [Burnley] in the north of England worked 20 or 25 years with this machine and has shown a lot about the pulse that was never known before and a great deal that was never even imagined by the physiologists. . . . You can see that [the patient] has a very irregular pulse and you can feel it now. In the long beats we can see that he has sometimes an extra-systole, and in addition the indi-

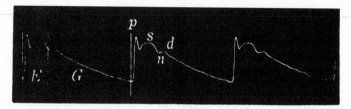

Sphygmogram of the radial pulse. The space E is the period of ventricular systole when the aortic valves are open ; the space G the period of ventricular diastole ; s is the pulse wave due to the ventricular systole ; n the aortic notch ; d the dicrotic wave ; and p a wave due to instrumental defect.

FIGURE 5. A normal sphygmogram. There is no time scale, but because the paper moved at a known, uniform speed, the time could be marked off with calipers. (From J. Mackenzie, *The Study of the Pulse*. Edinburgh: Young J. Pentland, 1902)

vidual beats vary somewhat in length so it looks as if he not only had some difference in conduction, but also some weakness in the contractility. The jugular pulse is also very curious. One place is probably an artifact, but it is so unusual looking it is quite hard to make out what it is. It looks like a little series of radial tracings, but of course, they have no business in that part of the tracing. . . . But the tracing itself does not show us what the disease is. That we have to get out by other means.

As for treatment of cardiac irregularity:

But a drug that a great many people look upon as highly useful in such a case is strychnine sulphate, although other people tell us it is of absolutely no use in the heart. They base their idea on the systolic blood pressure at the time. But I am strongly of the opinion that if you give strychnine you will find the heart getting regular more frequently than if you don't give strychnine. So I would give 1/30 of a grain every three or four hours, sometimes oftener.

Delerium Cordis

Dock had particular trouble understanding delerium cordis or absolute irregularity of the heart. Arthur Cushny, when he was studying cardiac irregularity caused by large doses of digitalis, had observed that auricular fibrillation results in ventricular irregularity similar to delerium cordis, and he produced it at will in dogs by rapid electrical stimulation of the auricles.[5] On December 29, 1901, Charles Wallis Edmunds, then an intern in the University Hospital, found absolute irregularity in a woman who had been operated upon by Reuben Peterson a few days before. He called Cushny, who was frequently consulted by clinicians. Cushny made sphygmographic tracings and diagnosed auricular fibrillation. Cushny and Edmunds soon showed their tracings at a meeting of the Ann Arbor Medical Club. They published their findings and interpretation in 1906 and again in 1907.[6] When electrocardiographic evidence became available, their interpretation was generally accepted.[7]

Up to 1907 at least, Dock did not agree with Cushny and Edmunds. In a long address to the State Medical Society of Wisconsin delivered on August 22, 1907, Dock described "fluttering of the heart" with irregular discharge of impulses from fibrillating auricles as a cause of occasional cardiac irregularity. As an explanation of perpetual arrhythmia, the possibility should be borne in mind, but the condition's elucidation is incomplete. Much later Dock's son William wrote: "Cushny fought, bled and died trying to convince him [George Dock] that delerium cordis was auricular fibrillation,—he [Dock] made lots of polygraph tracings but couldn't convince himself, did not trust the dogs."[8]

Valvular Lesions

Dock's students began their study of valvular disease by percussing to determine the size of the heart and by palpating to find the location of the apex beat. When Dock asked a student to describe the position of the apex beat, he said:

You never count from the clavicle; never count from the first rib, always from the second rib. Anybody who counts from the clavicle after the first semester will be conditioned. . . . So we take the median line or the edge of the sternum or the old fashioned landmark,—the nipple. Now of course it varies enormously in different patients, even in man. Of course in women we take an ideal nipple; but in man we take the patient's nipple.

Then the student auscultated and described what he found. Dock said:

[I]t requires the ability to listen to the heart without making a diagnosis, that is to listen to the murmurs, and to try to formulate the peculiarities of all the murmurs before you group the whole thing into a diagnosis.

If a student had difficulty telling whether a murmur was diastolic or systolic, Dock advised:

Timing the heart by the sounds when the heart is abnormal is a very faulty thing. You think the first is the second. Time the heart by the apex beat always if you can.

When a student could not tell whether a shock were systolic or diastolic, Dock instructed him to feel the carotid artery while he auscultated.

Many of the patients had aortic insufficiency and cardiac failure. In them, as Osler said: "On palpation the characteristic water-hammer or Corrigan pulse is felt. In the majority of instances the pulse wave strikes the finger forcibly with a quick jerking impulse, and immediately recedes or collapses. . . . the sphygmograph tracing is very characteristic. The high ascent, the sharp top, the quick drop in which the dicrotic notch and wave are very slightly marked."[9] Dock put it less elegantly: the sphygmogram goes straight up, then makes a number of jerks and comes straight down. Dock often showed sphygmograms taken from patients with aortic regurgitation. None has been preserved, but they must have looked like the ones Mackenzie published.[10]

There was also a capillary pulse: "We look at the patient's fingernails and what do we see? You see that when you first look at it you always wonder if it is not due to your own eyes. You see the color change and it

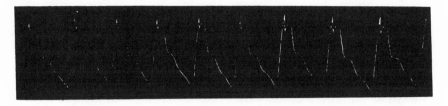

Pulse of slight aortic regurgitation with good heart-muscle.

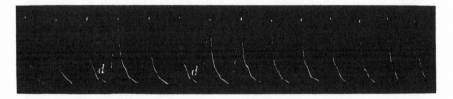

Pulse of extreme aortic regurgitation with great cardiac failure.

FIGURE 6. Two sphygmograms illustrating aortic regurgitation. (From J. Mackenzie, *The Study of the Pulse*. Edinburgh: Young J. Pentland, 1902)

has much the same effect as if you were winking. But if you look at it steadily, you will see there is really a capillary pulse there, showing the wave goes back and forth." Once the transcript said: "(Dr. Dock takes a towel and rubs the skin until it is red.) Dr. There is a capillary pulse, isn't there?"

Dock instructed his students to observe the delay between the apex beat and the appearance of the radial pulse in patients with aortic regurgitation. He may have been deceiving himself, for Mackenzie wrote: "there is no evidence of the extreme loss of time in the appearance of the radial pulse that the writers referred to [Flint, Balfour, Broadbent] have thought they detected."[11]

One man with water-hammer and capillary pulses also had a musical murmur. He was "A gentleman who goes around the country allowing people to examine his heart," and Dock said, with his insouciant disregard for accuracy in numbers, that he had been examined in three hundred medical schools and by thousands of medical students. Dock and his students heard the musical murmur, a blowing or whistling sound loudest over the lower part of the sternum, and in addition a soft diastolic murmur over the heart itself. Dock said the man had "Hibernian blood in him and had doubtless kissed the Blarney stone." He had been injured by a bayonet thrust, and Dock wondered whether the tricuspid valve had been lascerated. He thought the murmur might occur as a strong current of blood went over a sharp edge. At the end of the clinic the "class all examined," and one student passed the hat to collect fifteen cents from each of his classmates. Because there were 104 members of that fourth-year class, he could have collected $15.60.

Students were able to sort out murmurs resulting from multiple valvular lesions. Dock made the diagnosis of mitral regurgitation and probable aortic stenosis and insufficiency after a student had reported: "A systolic murmur at the apex, and also in the fourth intercostal space, just inside the nipple line, and I do not get that rumbling murmur. I can also hear a systolic murmur in the fourth intercostal space just to the left of the sternum and a sort of swishing sound after the second sound, and also a systolic murmur in the second i.c.s. I hear the two murmurs at the apex on the left side of the sternum, systolic and diastolic." Dock told the class to auscultate a patient with similar murmurs after the clinic, and on one occasion he told them to auscultate a dying patient because "It is very useful to have you all examine the patient so far as possible before the end does come."

Etiology of Valvular Disease

Dock attributed the double valvular disease he found in a long examination to rheumatism exacerbated by strain and overwork.

He has been working with his arms, working against an obstruction which would of course interfere with his breathing. He would probably produce an insufficiency of the mitral although it might have been on the right side of the heart. The latter part of his history is much more important, namely the history of rheumatism of an articular kind, and we know that would give him endocarditis, probably of the aortic valve.

Postrheumatic heart disease was a frequent finding in young patients. When Dock was examining a child in whom he made that diagnosis, he advised the class: "Hasten slowly with a child. Don't stare at him too much. Children are like animals in that respect. They can't stand the fixed gaze of human beings. Observe him without letting him know you are doing it." In this instance Dock found mitral insufficiency and regurgitation, and he said the prognosis was unfavorable; compensation will break before the child is twelve or fourteen. With an older student about to enter professional school Dock's prognosis was more optimistic:

> Very often a patient of this class asks about whether he is likely to drop dead suddenly. They ask because there is a widespread opinion among the laity that all people who drop dead have heart disease. Valvular disease is not a cause of sudden death. There is almost the same risk as being run over by a railroad train; but by taking reasonable care of himself and avoiding every strain and having his heart treated and cared for when it reaches conditions of relative weakness he can live a very long time.

The patient should not give up professional school. A patient of the same name graduated from law school two years later and another from engineering school four years later, but the identification of one or the other with the patient is uncertain.

Another young patient was not so fortunate. His rheumatism had moved from one joint to another; his heart was enlarged; and Dock thought he had both aortic and mitral regurgitation. He told the class:

> Here is an interesting therapeutic question. His father writes down that the two weeks are up and the boy ought to be well enough to come home; how he got the idea that it is a two week's case I don't understand. This illustrates how important it is to see that people understand that no definite time limit can be set. So I wrote the boy's father he was not well enough to try to go and certainly not well enough to stop treatment, and if he had to go home he ought to have treatment there. So the father writes that he is to come next Wednesday. Here is a man with his heart outside of him, yet the father would think of having him go off alone, carry-

ing a couple of grips, and starting on a long journey without much risk; but if anything happened to him he would blame the doctor for letting him go.

Dock told of a woman who had left against advice and who had caused great trouble by dying on the train with no identification about her.

Dock persuaded most medical visitors to substitute for him in giving a clinic. On May 24, 1905, "Dr. Frank Billings of Chicago," in town to address the county medical society, told the class about diagnosis of pneumococcal endocarditis, citing five of his own cases. He had brought some flasks with him, and he described how blood was drawn from a vein into the sterilized, partially evacuated flask containing culture medium. The cultures open "a new method of diagnosis." Treatment, however, was only palliative, for a positive finding was a death sentence. Billings said: "But it is a satisfaction to know what the diagnosis is even if you must tell the friends of the patient that he has got to die." Dock knew about the frequent misdiagnosis of malignant endocarditis, for he had written: "If endocarditis be mistaken for sepsis or for typhoid fever, the fatal issue is not so unexpected and the intractable course so inexplicable as when malarial disease is the diagnosis."[12]

Dock paraphrased Osler's comment that many men with aortic insufficiency had worshipped at the shrines of Mars and Venus,[13] but not before he had blamed the valvular disease of a Civil War veteran on endocarditis caused by pleuropneumonia the man had had more than thirty years earlier. In Dock's time at Michigan there was no serological test in the University Hospital for syphilis, but by 1903 he was attributing an aortic lesion to syphilis. Perhaps he was encouraged by his colleague Warthin, who was asserting that 25% of the hospital patients had syphilis.[14]

Aneurysm

The diagnosis of aneurysm of the aorta was first made by inspection. A thirty-seven-year-old woman had a bulging tumor under the inner third of the clavicle over the heart, greatest in the third interspace. Dock put a piece of paper on the tumor to show the class how it pulsated. A man presented with a harsh, low voice, a right palpebral slit much narrower than the left, a contracted right pupil that did not respond to light and pain over the neck and arm. When Dock asked what these suggested, a student immediately replied: aneurysm.

Dock demonstrated two methods of finding a tracheal tug. "The second method, and the best method is to stand behind the patient and have him stretch his neck; take the index fingers and grasp the crycoid cartilage and press upward. I certainly notice a slight tugging but you must exclude transmitted pulse from the arteries of the neck." A tracheal tug might be an unreliable sign of aneurysm. Dr. Sewall,[15] who had "examined enormous numbers of such [patients with tuberculosis] in Denver," had found tracheal tugging in patients with disease of the left pleura. Or a woman with enteroptosis and a "pendulous heart" that hangs not transversely but almost straight down may have a tracheal tug.

On January 16, 1900, students were told to look up the latest number of the *American Journal of Medical Sciences*, where someone had described tracheal diastolic shock as a sign of aortic aneurysm. The paper said: "This sign is, in brief, the transmission of the diastolic shock, originating at the same time as the closure of the aortic valves, through the aneurysm to the trachea, and manifest by a distinct, sharp impulse following the tracheal tug at the same interval as that between the apex-beat and the closure of the aortic segments."[16] In the same year the diagnosis was helped by fluoroscopy, for Dock scrawled at the end of the transcript for October 19, 1900: "X ray showed enormous enl. of heart, size of a man's hand, expanding ca 2 cm." At another time Dock showed two skiagraphs,[17] one of a normal individual and one with a bulge at the arch of the aorta.

The correct diagnosis might be missed, for an encysted empyema or a tumor might be mistaken for an aortic aneurysm. When a patient was referred to Dock from otolaryngology, Dock said:

He has a very interesting history and comes to us with the diagnosis already made. He has hoarseness and, on being examined by Dr. Cushman, was found to have paralysis of the left recurrent laryngeal nerve and was sent here as a suspected case of aneurysm of the aorta, and that is the way they are sometimes found. All are not always so fortunate in finding the diagnosis as this man. I once knew a man who had six different spray machines given him by six different doctors, one of them the author of a textbook on the Nose and Throat, and the whole six doctors had given him these sprays and machines on account of chronic laryngitis, when you could tell from the cough he had hardly anything else than this disease.

Dock said an aneurysm occurs rather late in life in men with a history of syphilis or alcoholism. Once: "When we look for an etiological factor, we find very simple conditions. He admits to a sore on the glans penis twenty years ago, and still shows the scar. But he has on the back of his neck so characteristic a leukoderma that as soon as I saw it I asked him if he ever had a sore, and it happens I was right."

Aneurysm is rare in women, and of one with no history of syphilis or alcoholism, Dock said:

That illustrates that severe muscular work is a very important factor in bringing on an aneurysm. Here is a woman who gives her occupation as housewife. What do you understand that to be? What sort of life do they lead?

STUDENT: Do you mean if they belong to the poorer classes?

DOCK: This woman might be said to belong to the richer classes, she is a farmer's wife, we might say from the financial standpoint, the middling class. How do you suppose such a woman spends her time? She certainly has a great deal of work to do. But suppose, besides doing housework, she does farm work, then what?

STUDENT: Then she does heavy work.

DOCK: It is important to realize that, because people in this country have an idea that women do not do that kind of work. In Europe, I have seen them carrying hods up four or five story buildings, with a load of mortar and brick; and have seen them harnessed with a cow, while another woman worked the plow. [This patient] took her part in the hay harvest, and has been doing that ever since she was married, barring, perhaps, the time she was operated, and she was lucky to have escaped that long. Dr. Peterson had a case in which he advised a woman to have an operation; but the husband objected because his wife was a good hand and had to work, he said; and rather than lose the time being operated he let her keep on half sick.

An aneurysm might be "wired" so that clots formed around the wires, or a patient might benefit from potassium iodide whether or not he had syphilis. Dock had seen one aneurysm shrink so much that the man could pass a life insurance examination. Otherwise, the patient must lead a simple life and "if constipated by all means avoid straining at stool." But "such a thing may stop life at any minute. You may see your patient, find him improved and cheerful, and before you get out of the house he may be dead."

Measuring Blood Pressure

On October 27, 1903, just after Cook had described his "practical instrument for routine use" in measurement of arterial blood pressure,[18] Dock first told his students the results of such a measurement made on his wards. Thereafter, Dock used the Cook instrument, the Stanton one or the Janeway variation.[19] He recommended Janeway's book on the clinical study of blood pressure.[20] With all these instruments, systolic pressure was estimated as the pressure at which the radial pulse disappeared or appeared as the cuff was inflated or deflated. Dock said that no machine gave reliable measurement of diastolic pressure, but diastolic pressure could be estimated as the pressure at which the greatest oscillation of the mercury occurred. In 1908 he said he was not familiar with the Erlanger instrument,[21] which allowed reasonably accurate measurement of diastolic pressure.

Dock and his staff enjoyed comparing the tension estimated by the time-honored method of feeling the pulse with that determined with a sphygmomanometer: "All take pleasure in guessing the pressure before we take it, and sometimes we have good guesses, but every now and then we have an experience that makes us think it is all guessing. Here we guessed 130 and 140. All were very far from it."

On December 13, 1907, Dock guessed that the pressure in a patient

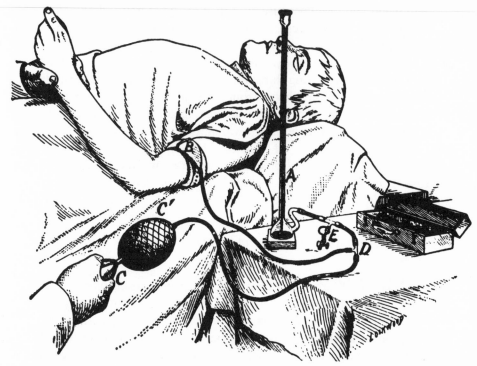

FIGURE 7. Cook's method of measuring systolic blood pressure. (From T. Janeway, *The Clinical Study of Blood-pressure*. New York: D. Appleton and Company, 1904)

with abdominal pulsations was over 150 and possibly 170. He sent for a sphygmomanometer.

We will let Dr. Van [Zwaluwenburg] get it without mentioning what it is, and then we will let Mr. Anderson take it and see what we get. This is undoubtedly one of the most useful additions to mechanical diagnosis that we have ever had. Do you know the principle of it? What you do is this: You feel the pulse; then we shut off the blood in the artery by blowing the bag full of air. Now at the point where the blood overcomes the air, of course, is the systolic pressure, that is, the force necessary to get the blood past the obstruction. Now as the mercury goes above the point the pulse will disappear. What you want to do is to carefully feel the radial and note when you lose the pulse, and then as the mercury drops you feel it again. We will get Dr. Van to write his down and then you call out where you get it and see where they match. 142, 130, 137. It proves one of the points I made before, that it is hard to get. But here is a very interesting thing, although the systolic pressure isn't very high I should say the diastolic very likely is. I get the change of pulse about 95, that is the pulse gets smaller, which is looked upon when you get it clearly as evidence of a minimum pulse.

Obviously measurement of blood pressure was not yet routine on the wards.

Arteriosclerosis and Hypertension

Before blood pressure could be measured, hypertension was detected by the nature of the pulse. Osler wrote of the high-tension pulse of arteriosclerosis: "The pulse wave is slow in its ascent, enduring, subsides slowly, and in the intervals between beats the vessel remains full and firm. It may be difficult to obliterate the pulse, and the firmest pressure on the radial or temporal artery may not be sufficient to annihilate the pulse wave beyond the point of pressure."[22] Osler quoted Cohnheim on the *essential* nature of hypertension in arteriosclerosis; high arterial pressure is necessary to force blood through the sclerotic renal vessels.

When Dock could measure systolic pressure, he wrote that "[t]he recognition of the earliest stages of arteriosclerosis is only beginning to assume a practical character. By the use of instruments for measuring blood pressure . . . it will be possible to put this subject on a more definite basis than at present."[23] In that paper he reported the case of a boy with acute nephritis whose pressure was "170 to 190 mm measured with Cook's Riva-Rocci instrument." In the latest stages of arteriosclerosis, Dock said, systolic pressure may reach 240.

Dock attempted to explain the relations among arteriosclerosis, hypertension and renal disease. In 1904 he wrote that "the importance of hypertension in causing vascular changes [in the kidney] is now well recognized."[24] When a patient with arteriosclerosis but with little albumin in his urine was presented, Dock told the class:

That [minimal albuminuria] is a very curious and important fact,—if he has arteriosclerosis the kidney is almost certainly to be affected in time but the liver isn't. The blood supply is entirely different, i.e., the kidney has to stand a large quantity of any kind of urine going through it. But these same things may not affect the liver; whereas if there are certain toxic substances in the abdominal cavity, with access to the portal veins, then the liver is likely to be affected.

On the other hand,

[a] chronic nephritis, either interstitial or parenchymatous, in a person with previously healthy blood vessels, may cause arteriosclerosis by retention of injurious substances, which act either on the vessel walls or cause reflex spasm.[25]

Arteriosclerotic changes in the vessel walls can be seen in the retina. When a patient with severe albuminuria, dyspnea and edema of the legs was examined, the student responsible reported he had seen the patient's eye grounds. The discs, the vessels and the macula were normal, he said, but, "[o]utside of that there are diffuse points of recent hemorrhage. . . . At other points there are black spots of older hemorrhage, and at other points there are almost white areas, indicating probably atrophy of the choroid or of the retina." The student's diagnosis was "retinitis albuminurica." Fleming Carrow, the professor of ophthalmology, in whose clinic the student had examined the eye grounds, had said the patient would last about six months. The patient should avoid meat, for meat throws more work on the kidneys and increases arterial tension. Otherwise, there is no treatment.

Diagnosis with Roentgen Rays

Shortly after the discovery of X rays became generally known early in 1896, Will Herdman, Michigan's professor of electrotherapeutics, rigged up a Crookes tube and made skiagraphs of a bullet in the hand, of one in the collar bone, of a needle in the foot and of a dislocated shoulder.[26] From early in 1900 at the latest, fluoroscopy and skiagraphy were available in the University Hospital under the direction of Herdman and his assistant, Vernon J. Willey. After Herdman died late in 1905, Willey remained in charge of roentgenology until after Dock left Michigan.

There was no formal teaching of roentgenology in Dock's time, and Dock had to explain to the students that a skiagraph represents the patient as if he were facing you. One technique was to make a tracing on the fluorescent screen, and when Dock showed one such he said:

[It] looks wider in the tracing, and I think we can explain it by the action of the perspective on the heart. It shows one of the weak points of the x-ray for topographical illustration, and there is simply no way of getting out of the difficulty. Pieces of apparatus have been devised using the diaphragm, and various machines that put up a system of markers, but none of them are practically useful."

Dock was referring to the "orthodiagraph."[27] There was one in the University Hospital after, but probably not during, Dock's time in Ann Arbor.

Dock compared the results of percussion with a tracing made using the fluoroscope.

A student who had seen his patient twice daily made the diagnosis of pericardial effusion. Dock said he should have seen the patient more often, and he asked for more evidence to support the diagnosis. When they examined a skiagraph of the heart:

STUDENT: It is enlarged on both sides, isn't it?

DOCK: And what else?

STUDENT: It looks very distinct.

DOCK: Well, what has that to do with it?

STUDENT: I don't know whether that would show the motion on the skiagraph or not.

DOCK: Yes, that is a good point; just enlarge that.

STUDENT: (Stenographer couldn't hear.)

DOCK: That is quite true. Especially one taken with such a long exposure. Your point is well made, one must be struck by the sharpness of the edge, and even if taken in one second his heart must have made at least two movements and there would be a little shadow along there, and it does not appear to be so, and what would that make you think? That there was an effusion there so that the sac was not being moved by the movement of the heart but filled with a fluid that gives it this shape and prevents the movement.

Treatment of Heart Failure; Dock's Twenty Drugs

Most of the patients with valvular disease had one degree or another of what Dock called *incompensation*. An exception was a girl of ten with mitral regurgitation and a defect in the septum. Dock told her mother that the child would never be free of her lesion; no medicine would remove that. He told the class that she could retain her compensation for a long time but that it was likely to run out during puberty.

Every year Dock drilled his students in the diagnosis of heart failure. First, there was cyanosis. It might be only in the ears or it might extend to the hands and feet. Dock said of one sallow patient with widespread cyanosis: "He has the yellow and blue color which is not so much a cause for rejoicing as on the football field." Michigan colors are maize and blue, and those were the days of Fielding Yost's "point-a-minute" teams. Edema of the legs extending to the scrotum or labia was observed, and sometimes the circumference of the leg was measured. Patients with failure had dyspnea, and many were orthopneic. Dock pointed out how one was struggling to sit up rather than lie flat on the examining table. Dimensions of the enlarged heart were carefully determined by percussion, and fine, crackling rales resulting from pulmonary edema were heard by auscultation.

If a patient were ambulatory, he might be given graded exercise. Dock said: "The celebrated Ertel cure for heart disease practiced in Germany where patients are given a prescription for walking, telling them how many degrees of elevation to go and how many kilo[meter]s distance." When a student said he would regulate a patient's life, Dock told him: "When you regulate her life, like a good many others, you will find it easier to talk about than to see that it gets regulated." Of a patient who had fainted several times while defecating and had died at stool, Dock said:

> The average individual when he comes to the hospital and is asked to use a bed pan says he can't. If you ask him if he ever tried it, he will say no. Anybody can use a bed pan with very little trouble. Usually one trial is enough. In the case of the individual who is likely to faint, he should never be allowed to sit up because defecating very often is an exhausting process.

For that patient, the outcome would have been the same anyway.

Of a patient with dyspnea, Dock said:

> He wants to be by the open window to get fresh air. The air he gets in the window is not very different from the air in the room; but it gives him a feeling of refreshment. The same feeling can be helped to a greater extent by giving him oxygen. Oxygen in cylinders is easily obtained because dentists get it to give with laughing gas.

But a few whiffs of oxygen every half hour are useless.

Dock has discarded bleeding. He said of a saloon keeper with cachexia, orthopnea, cyanosis, an aortic murmur and edema:

> We might bleed him half a pint. He might become very much better, breathe more easily, express himself as feeling well, and again in half an hour, he would be worse than before. We might bleed him again. He would become still worse and so it goes.

Alternatively:

> Or in these anemic days we can bleed a man into his own blood vessels. Do you know how to do that? It referred to the use of [nitroglycerine] or nitrite; the idea being that this dilated blood vessels and lessened the resistance in the circulation and the heart worked more easily. It is just the same as bleeding; instead of making the blood too small for the vessels it made the vessels too large for the blood.

In addition to nitroglycerine, Dock used digitalis, strychnine, and diuretin for patients in failure.

Every year Dock gave a more or less formal lecture on therapeutics. In 1900 he began by saying:

> What I want to point out to the beginner is that it is possible to get along extremely well without the knowledge of hundreds of various kinds of drugs. This is especially true after you pass certain State Examining Boards. In some states they ask about certain drugs that nobody ever heard of. In New York, for instance there were drugs spoken of which Drs. Abel and Cushny and a good many practicing physicians had never heard of. One young man who passed the examination with credit asked why they had those in. They said they had to ask a certain number of questions and had not enough to go around, so they had some dummy questions that they put in they did not expect anyone to know about them, but had to keep up appearances.

Dock said he was guided

> by the expression we sometimes see quoted, which appears to come from the early part of the 17th century, that the young physician has 20 remedies for every disease but the older one has 20 remedies for all diseases. It occurred to me a long time ago that perhaps one could find 20 drugs that could simplify the practice of medicine.

Here is the list Dock gave in 1900:

1. Opium and its derivatives
2. Arsenic
3. Potassium iodide
4. Quinine
5. Digitalis
6. Strychnine
7. Salicylic acid
8. Potassium bromide
9. Ammonium chloride
10. Iron
11. Atropine or belladonna
12. Hypnotics; sulphonal or chloral
13. Phenacetin
14. Calomel
15. Bismuth
16. Nitrites; nitroglycerine
17. Alcohol
18. Ipecac
19. Potassium acetate
20. Balsam

The list differed in detail from year to year. Sometimes it included mercury, and in 1905 Dock substituted saline diuretics for potassium acetate, eliminated alcohol and added turpentine. Dock's use of cardiac drugs will be described here and his use of other drugs in the appropriate place.

Dock said digitalis is more important than any other cardiac stimulant, and he wanted a preparation that had been tested physiologically. Physicians in the University Hospital preferred to use a freshly prepared infusion of English rather than of German leaves, for the English were usually the purer. There were many preparations of derivatives on the market, and all claimed to have no side effects. Dock was skeptical of the claims; he said the preparations were simply more expensive.

The proper dose of the tincture of digitalis was 20 drops three times a day. This might be too large, and the patient would have "what we call a digitalis pulse. The pulse is stronger than in an ordinary individual. In addition it is full and slow." Then the dose was to be reduced to 10 drops for two days and skipped for three days.

Sometimes Dock had a student write a prescription for digitalis on the blackboard, and when he asked the student how the dose was to be measured Dock said: "The best way is to look at the patient's teaspoon and make a guess as to how much it contains or take it out and measure it, but with medicine you want to give in small doses it is just as safe to drop it with a dropper or from the bottle, and suppose the patient does drop 17 instead of 15, there is no very great harm done. In practical therapeutics we give approximate doses."

Dock gave strychnine to most patients with heart failure. He preferred large doses, and he said most physicians did not give enough. For a patient in severe failure Dock prescribed 1/30 grain four times a day, given hypodermically for eight days, and after digitalis was stopped strychnine was continued indefinitely as a heart tonic.

Dock's enthusiasm for strychnine was not shared by Arthur Cushny, who said: "Strychnine seems to be of benefit in some cases of heart disease and is often supposed to have a direct effect upon that organ. Any improvement which may be produced by it, however, must be attributed to the constriction of the vessels, and the indication for its use would seem to be low blood pressure."[28] James Mackenzie was even more forthright. In discussing "cardiac tonics" he wrote:

The most popular remedy of this class is strychnine, or some preparation of nux vomica. I have carefully sought for its special effect upon the heart and found none. When I enquired into the evidence for its supposed good effect, I found it was practically all clinical, and clinical evidence endows the drug with the most diverse properties. . . . The evidence that shows a drug to possess the property of exciting the sluggish and of soothing the excited, of raising the low pressure and relieving the high, speaks more for unreasoning faith in the drug than for the beneficial properties of the drug itself.[29]

By 1908 Dock had become defensive about his continued use of strychnine, and he asserted his faith in his own clinical experience to validate its continued use.

An edematous patient was given diuretin.

DOCK: That is the name of a diuretic, but is that all it does? What is it? You ought to have looked that up. Did you ever hear of it before in Dr. Cushny's book? Well, what is it, Chapman?

STUDENT: I don't know that I can state exactly.

DOCK: Well, do you know approximately or inexactly? Chase, Chapman, Beekes?

STUDENT: I thought it was a caffeine compound.

DOCK: What is it, Morehouse?

STUDENT: Equal parts of theobromine and sodium salicylate.

DOCK: That is the combination.

As for dosage:

DOCK: It has always been my intention to have the dose on the charts to show the quantity of the effective agent the patient gets; for example, on the chart it should be, "Diuretin, grains 15, every three hours." It is quite possible that the dose of the vehicle is there, and that is bad—well, it is marked "two drachms." Why in the world is that? We have a standing order in the pharmacy to have the formula on the bottle, because students can best learn about amounts in dosage practically.

A patient with mitral insufficiency, cyanosis, edematous legs and swollen abdomen was given digitalis, strychnine and diuretin. Eleven days later she no longer coughed; signs of exudate and congestion of the lungs had disappeared; and she had lost twenty-two pounds.

No matter how severe the failure, Dock said: "To give up a patient in this condition is a very serious fault in practice. One has to be perfectly understood by the patient and relatives and tell them that complete recovery is out of the question. . . . Doctors knowing the serious prognosis that is in store for them, are usually much worse than other patients."

Coronary Artery Disease

A student presented the history of a large, robust man with traces of cyanosis in ears and fingertips, a slight beating in the jugular fossa, and respiratory frequency "a little too rapid for a man who is perfectly well."

STUDENT: He complains of paroxysms of pain over the cardiac region, and at this time he has difficulty taking a long breath. This shortness of breath lasts for two minutes and he becomes faint, and after the pain which lasts from two seconds to a minute or two he can take a full breath. Then he has pains in his legs and arms of the character of sharp shooting pains and radiating out—he held his fingers this way—and at the end there is numb feeling, and his hands and feet during the attack are numb and swollen.

DOCK: Well, what do you think about that?

STUDENT: Those attacks are suggestive of angina pectoris.

DOCK: What do you understand by it?

STUDENT: Some theories say . . .

DOCK: I am not talking about the theory; but do you mean by that a distinct definite disease like locomotor ataxia, or a disease, for example, like hyperchlorhydria?

STUDENT: I think it is more of a symptom.

DOCK: Then the next question is, Is it always the same kind of symptom, that is, does every angina pectoris case act like every other?

STUDENT: No, I think not.

DOCK: Then the next question is, What do you mean as regards causation? Can we tell from the history of pain whether the patient has one or the other of a large number of organic diseases of the circulation?

STUDENT: I think we can.

DOCK: Then how do you tell?

STUDENT: You get the paroxysmal pain as if the heart was in a vice.

DOCK: Did he devise that simile himself or did somebody suggest it to him. (To patient): How did you get the idea?

PATIENT: I thought of it myself.

DOCK: What is the matter with the man's heart? Can we ever find out?

STUDENT: I could not in this case. In some cases where there is marked arteriosclerosis we think of sclerosis of the coronaries.

DOCK: Is it possible to have sclerosis of the coronaries and not anywhere else?

STUDENT: I think so.

DOCK: Oh yes, that is so common that it would be the first thing we think of; not that he had angina from dilatation or aneurysm or pericardial adhesions, but that he had it from coronary artery disease. . . . What would you say was the most likely explanation of the attacks of angina?

STUDENT: I thought it was due to ischaemia of the heart muscle.

Dock prescribed nitroglycerine, 1/200 of a grain every two hours, although nitroglycerine gave this patient a headache. Some relatives ought to be told that he is the sort of man who might die suddenly. If he has any important business, that ought to be looked after. The most important thing is to regulate his life. Almost any function, eating, defecating, might bring on a fatal attack.

This patient was presented on March 27, 1908, but patients with similar problems had been presented earlier. It would be surprising if Dock's students were not fully aware of the diagnosis of coronary artery disease during life. Dock must have repeated to them the essence of the lecture "Some Notes on the Coronary Arteries," which he had given in Buffalo in 1906. The *Medical and Surgical Reporter* had published the lecture and ascribed it to George Doch [*sic*]. In the lecture Dock reviewed the history of the recognition of coronary artery disease during life.

The most illustrious example of this is furnished by the oft-cited case of John Hunter. The acute Jenner correctly diagnosed the calcification of the coronary arteries and referred to them the anginal attacks of his friend and teacher. Parry, too, in several cases was able to make similar predictions, verified post-mortem. On the whole, such cases were not common enough to soon make an impression on the profession as a whole, and it is not surprising that later writers allowed the subject to escape them.[30]

It had not escaped Dock, for he concluded by presenting four cases of his own.[31]

DISEASES OF THE LUNGS, EXCLUDING TUBERCULOSIS

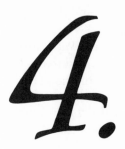

IN ASTHMA, DOCK SAID, DYSPNEA
is not continuous: "The breathing grows more and more labored until
the patient seemingly cannot breathe at all and at the height of this
dyspnea by coughing or by some sudden exercise the patient suddenly
becomes easy of breath and the attack subsides." A student questioned
by Dock about asthma replied:

> The general idea of asthma is that it is rather a symptom than a
> disease.
>
> DOCK: That is a very good idea. One must go through the symp-
> toms of asthma and ask the patient about them; but there is one
> thing we have to think about asthma and that it is a very unsatis-
> factory term applied to many dyspnoeic diseases, and first of all
> heart disease.

When Dock questioned another student about a patient with dyspnea,
mitral regurgitation and dilatation of the right heart, the student said:

> She gives a history of attacks of asthma.
>
> DOCK: Is that idiopathic asthma, that is, neurotic asthma or
> the result of cardiac lesion or does it come from the nasal septum
> or what? Even if she had nervous asthma that would be likely to
> come on most at night, but isn't that true of cardiac asthma? Yes,
> it is likely to come on at any time, especially if people have over-
> strained the heart, but on the other hand it is highly characteristic
> of cardiac dyspnea the patients have at night because the heart be-
> gins to work less; if in addition she has been eating freely and had
> her stomach full of food and had indigestion, which she would

68

very likely have from her cardiac condition, then that would still further increase the pressure of the abdominal organs upon the diaphragm and then she would have asthma for that.

Otherwise, one must look for a focus. Dr. Canfield, the professor of otolaryngology, said that a twenty-nine-year-old farmer with asthmatic attacks since childhood had a spur in his nose. Dock said:

> But still the first thing to do is to begin at the beginning and remove the respiratory anomalies as fast as we can find them. Here is a place where we never give medicine unless we catch him in a paroxysm. But still the first thing to do is to find the anomaly; in this case, take the spur and operate on that and the turbinate and operate on that, and then if he has adenoids, get rid of those, and all the other possible sources. Then take the constipation and dilate the stomach and treat those and when he has an attack, then make careful searches for still other foci of infection.

Of another patient with asthma Dock said that she had a disease especially influenced by financial conditions; the best remedy is a change of climate. Otherwise she should have a light diet and large doses of potassium iodide, 20 grains three times a day after meals, best taken in milk. She could inhale turpentine vapor during an attack. A counterirritant would help: croton oil or a mixture of turpentine and vinegar.

Dyspnea and Bronchitis

At the beginning of a year Dock told his students they must begin to notice the signs of respiratory diseases. A student should have seen that his patient had clubbed fingers with broad, short nails, unlike those of tuberculosis, which are longer and curved like the beak of a bird. A man's posture told the story, Dock continued: "Hasn't he the appearance of a man who is holding his shoulders up? He holds his shoulders very high, and that is a change we find very often in thoracic disease where there is difficulty on inspiration. You should notice all characteristics of breathing aside from rales, and particularly notice the length of inspiration and expiration." Of another patient:

STUDENT: During inspiration he seems to experience a great amount of pain and you notice a marked movement in the epigastrium.

DOCK: What sort of movement?

STUDENT: It is a kind of pulling in of the tissues.

DOCK: We have a technical term for "pulling in." Instead of using Anglo Saxon we use a Latin derivative for such things. We call it retraction.

In contrast, a patient with a chronic cough and a hyperresonant, barrel chest had prolonged expiration.

STUDENT: There might be emphysema from this chronic condition.

DOCK: How?

STUDENT. From the distention which follows chronic coughing.

DOCK: What causes the distention?

STUDENT: Expelling air from the lungs so violently breaks down the lung tissue, and then when the air comes in again, it would fill the space that has been left.

DOCK: Do you mean the air rushing in does the damage? If a person ran out of the house, would there be a danger of a room being crushed out from the inside?

STUDENT: I think that some of the tissues are clogged with mucus, and expelling causes this condition.

DOCK: How?

STUDENT: The [contraction?] of the thoracic muscles and the diaphragm produces pressure in the lungs, and if the exit is closed, then that causes the condition.

DOCK: Now you are getting at it.

A patient with a chronic cough might produce 400 to 500 cc of sputum every day. Dock said that patients could go without coughing a long time, but "as soon as they get in that position they begin to cough, and then they find that they can empty the whole thing at once, get themselves into a curious position and then gulp up or spit up 1/2 pint of sputum." Dock often passed around sputum for students to examine, but sometimes he did not. "I guess we had better not send this specimen around because it may be a little too much. [But another was worse.] You could hardly get near him." Once a dish of sputum Dock said:

> That is a very interesting specimem of sputum, sputum having a thin watery mucous basis and having in it rather long or some-times rounded or irregular masses of yellowish color, having greater consistency than the rest, and then we can see on the slide which I pass around on the book because it offers a good back-ground for the sputum, you can see some of those characteristic long pieces that have been taken out of the sputum and can be put on the glass. It may not strike you as being distinctly spiral but yet they are very good sputum spirals.

Dock was asking students to see Curshmann's spirals, coiled mucinous fibrils sometimes seen in the sputum of patients with bronchial asthma, chronic bronchitis and even pneumonia. They were thought to indicate desquamative catarrh of the bronchi and alveoli.[1] Dock said that the pearls Laënnec had described were really spirals; Laënnec had not spread them out to show their spiral structure. Dock said: "If you fasten a stick to sputum at one end and then blow along it it will form spirals such as we find here."

Elastic tissue or tubercle bacilli had not been found in any of these specimens of sputum, but Dock as always told his students not to rely on a singly negative result. Keep on staining samples until you are sure.

A student suggested that cod liver oil is the appropriate treatment for a child with a chronic cough; the oil would sooth the membranes of the mouth. Dock replied: "Did you ever taste cod liver oil? Most people don't consider it soothing. The cod liver oil idea is passing away, partly because there is a famine at present, most of the cod liver oil being made of cottonseed oil, flavored to taste bad." Instead, Dock would give a mild expectorant in syrup of wild cherry. "There is one drug that is very useful in such cases and that is strychnia. It is a useful stimulant of the whole respiratory apparatus." On other occasions Dock prescribed a mixture of potassium iodide, 10 grains of ammonium bromide, 6 drops of tincture of belladonna and 5 grains of ammonium chloride, repeated every hour. A patient with a loud, high-pitched cough that was extremely painful not only to her but to anybody that had to hear it was given 1/4 grain of heroin every three hours. The heroin, or alternatively codeine, was given hypodermically. Dock said:

> I was going to speak somewhat on the matter of hypodermics, and we might as well seize the opportunity now. In order to give hypodermic injections it is necessary to have a proper syringe. The modern hypodermics with screw attachments for the needle are impossible to keep clean. 15 years ago nobody ever saw a hypodermic needle with a screw in it; however, if you insist, you can get your druggist to get one with a ground joint. The needle should always be kept clean. It must be washed out with warm water after using it. As a matter of fact, in the good old days before we knew we ought to keep our hands clean and other people's skin clean, I have seen a good many hypodermics given by a good many dirty doctors to dirty patients and rarely have seen any abscesses. If [the syringe] has leather packing, it should be washed out if used with quinine or other corrosive substances. It is not always necessary to boil the syringe. You can boil the needle. The needle should be kept sharp to avoid pain. They can be kept sharp by rubbing them occasionally on an oil stone, a thing that every doctor should have in his office. The usual method is to pinch up the skin, stick the needle in parallel to the surface and then inject into the subcutaneous tissues. Why it should be given there, I have never been able to find out. Any fluid will be taken up just as well in muscular tissue as in the subcutaneous. There is an idea that if you inject into solid tissue, you run the risk of getting into a vein. Out of millions of hypodermics every week, we practically never hear of it affecting the veins directly. There is so much difficulty trying to get the veins for various purposes, it is easy to understand that in the ordinary use you do not get into the veins. The biceps, or outer part of the forearm is a very good place. I once worked out an experiment in injecting quinine and found that the patients preferred to have injections in the forearm to any other part of the body except the buttocks. Having it in, you inject the fluid steadily. We draw it out and then work the hand over the place a few minutes.

Dock said the thorax of a woman with a cough sounded "not unlike a pigeon loft," and he had his students listen to her as well as to all others. When he used one patient to demonstrate the difference between a friction rub and rales, the sound disappeared while he was listening. "So you mustn't draw the conclusion that your first listening was wrong." When one student described what he heard, Dock said to another student:

What do you think of the description that has just been given? What is the matter with it?

STUDENT: It is not complete. He did not describe what kind of breathing on the left for one thing. He paid too much attention to the rales and not enough to describing the changes in the respiratory conditions.

DOCK: Yes, the reason being that the rales are more uncertain of interpretation than the other sounds. Suppose the patient's rales disappear during the night, as they not infrequently do; then you will have to start all over again.

Dock defended his practice of having one student criticize another by saying that a doctor must retain his self-possession under all circumstances. He might as well begin to learn that while in medical school.

A student said that rales are made by "congestion of the lungs and separation of the small bronchi." Dock scorned the answer.

When a person inspires we know very well that the air does not rush immediately into the alveoli. It goes into the bronchi, but from them it is taken up by diffusion. It is not as if the air got all in and out again and the lung wall collapsed as a door will shut when there is a draft outward through the house; there are cilia in the winding passages and as they move slightly they give a crackling or snapping sound. They don't need to move very far or snap very hard.

Pneumonia

A patient demonstrated in the clinic had pain so that he could not lie on his right side.

PATIENT: I was spitting up a substance that looked like pounded liver. I felt as if I had to pass my checks in the next Saturday night.

DOCK: That isn't a bad description of what?

STUDENT: Lobar pneumonia.

DOCK: I think there is another thing you ought to see. You have to be able to see it easily because when you see it at home it is usually in an alcove if there is an alcove about the house and the alcove is usually darkened so as to keep the air out as well as the light.

STUDENT: I think there is cyanosis.

DOCK: That is the idea.

Dock showed the sputum of a patient with pneumonia:

Are you through looking at it, Brookhart? What do you see there? Don't pass anything until you are sure you know all about it.

STUDENT: It has two distinct colors, a reddish color and also a yellow, and on top of that a white foam.

DOCK: How about the consistency of it?

STUDENT: It sticks to the cup.

DOCK: Yes, it is rather tenacious; not as tenacious as you sometimes say about sputum, for example, it doesn't stick to the sides of the cup; it doesn't stick to his lips, but still after it gets into the bottom of the cup it keeps its original shape; it does not float out like a watery mucous sputum but is rather tenacious or gelatinous; and the color, as you probably see, is both red and yellow and if you had seen it before you would have seen that it had a slight reddish yellow color and it might occur to one that the yellow was really a red yellow, the color that iron rust gets when it is mixed with other material.

A microscope was always available, and students examined preparations of sputum containing "Diplococci, probably pneumococci, also some other germs, streptococci probably." They also made blood counts, and they found "a leucocytosis of 25000. All these things make it quite certain that he had croupous pneumonia." In 1907 Dock could add: "Then we might get a blood culture and then work the opsonins with reference to pneumonia and other things."

When he auscultated a patient with pneumonia, a student said he heard large, moist rales.

> DOCK: What would you say they sound like? Did they sound like hair rubbed between the fingers?
>
> STUDENT: They were much larger than that.
>
> DOCK: Did they sound like crackling in a flame? It seems to me there is a comparison more like it, and that is crackling a piece of rather stiff paper.

Another student found weak fremitus and said that that condition suggests consolidation of the lung. Dock replied that consolidation increases fremitus. "But a more common cause is a voice too weak to cause vocal fremitus." Dock told him that

> if you listen over the back you will get a sound that must strike you as tubular, that is, it has a concentrated sound, a sound that you can imitate by making certain movements with your mouth. But put your mouth in this position to pronounce the sounds of "Ha" in a whispering voice, say "ha, he, hi, ho," you can imitate the sounds of blowing breathing. Get your tongue clear from saliva, otherwise saliva will make rales. Once you hear the breathing in pneumonia and you will be struck by the peculiar tubular sound, even over the trachea you will not remember having heard such a thing.

Dock sent students downstairs to the ward in groups of four to hear "coarse liquid probably so-called redux rales that appear in pneumonia when softening begins."

There were babies with pneumonia. Dock remarked:

> When you auscult a baby, a baby old enough to take notice of things, it is a great deal better never to auscult in front, especially with a stethoscope. Because if you go to work with something shiny like a stethoscope the baby will begin to cry so that you can't

do anything. Sometimes it is better to listen with the ear. You can auscult it in the back while it is in the nurse's or the mother's arms, and the child will not know what is going on. If you begin by hitting it, which is the way it looks on percussion, it will cry all the time. It is not always a disadvantage when the baby cries when you are ausculting. When it cries it takes deep breaths [and that allows judgment of transmission of the voice].

Every now and then a patient described in the afternoon clinic had postoperative pneumonia. One was a five-year-old girl who had had a mastoid operation. Dock had removed 150 cc of pus from her chest, and he thought the chest might have to be drained by incision. He said:

> The greatest trouble with such cases is that they are allowed to go without physical examination. These cases occur frequently. I have seen two in the last two weeks where both cases had gotten over attacks diagnosed as pneumonia, getting along much better, but not getting entirely well. In one case the child was treated for stomach disease and in the other nothing was done, but in neither case was the patient examined. So the thing to do is to examine very frequently after improvement because a child with pneumonia usually gets over the pneumonia, but the danger comes from complications in the pleura.

Another patient was referred from the ear clinic with a fever of 106° and double pneumonia. "The long operation and anaesthesia were simply a life-saving operation, and the risk that these could be stood had simply to be taken. That is, we don't tell people every time we operate on them that they run the risk of getting pneumonia, but it is always there, so we always tell people that an operation may be dangerous." All patients in a series of fifty cases had survived, and Dock attributed their recovery to the treatment they had received. This patient died.

Treatment of Pneumonia

Sometimes pneumonia was aborted. In 1904 a patient had been sent to the University Hospital with a diagnosis of pneumonia. His temperature was normal after three days, and the leucocyte count was down to 7,000 from 21,000.

DOCK: What aborted it?

STUDENT: The treatment he received here.

DOCK: That is a good way to look at it. It speaks well for your charitable heart. There is nothing more natural than to think his care has been the cause of his change. If you flatter yourself too much for aborting a case, then you will be blamed if any run over. Although there are people who believe they have methods by which they can abort the process in the lungs, the fact is that pneumonia aborts itself.

Dock said he had been raised in the heroic school of treatment of pneumonia. He had put on fly plasters 9×5 to 12×18 inches, sometimes on both sides, "drawing literally quarts of serum." He had never seen it do any good.[2] "Poultice has never shortened the disease by a minute."

We do not know of any drug that will stop a forming pneumonia. We do not know of any serum that would do that, although serum is being worked on [in 1901]. What is the use of giving drugs if they do not do any good? . . . When we say a disease is self-limited we mean a disease that has a tendency to subside, even if nothing is done for the patient. Pneumonia of course gets well, but as far as I have been able to discover the idea that the disease is self-limited came out when first definitely demonstrated that pneumonia cases would get well without the strenuous treatment to which they were subjected at that time. About the middle of the last century the patient with pneumonia had very strong treatment applied to him. They were almost invariably bled, almost always salivated, and depressed with tartar emetic. It was shown by taking pneumonia patients and giving a series of them this treatment and the other series no treatment at all that they would get well about the same time.

The best treatment is provided by a cool-headed nurse and consists of calomel at the start, digestible food at short intervals, plenty of water and scrupulous care of the mouth. If the patient is a baby, give it a bath at 90°. That makes the baby struggle and improve the breathing. Digitalis might be given if the patient is cyanotic, and "KI and ammonium chloride would do no harm." Otherwise, let the patient alone. Do not give antipyretics, and do not bleed the patient. "Very few people who talk about the beauty of bleeding in pneumonia practice it. The average general practitioner who sees his patients in the early stages rarely tries it."

A doctor had told his patient to take whisky, for whisky strengthens the lungs. Dock did not use alcohol for pneumonia or for anything else. He cited his experience in the industrial district of Philadelphia where many patients were alcoholics.

> Perhaps I ought to enlarge a little on the subject of alcohol because the friend I quoted [on digitalis] makes the following statement. He says that in the beginning a patient should not be given alcohol unless he has been a hard drinker; then he should be given alcoholic drinks in order to prevent delerium tremens. That is a plausible idea, an idea held by every drinking man. But anybody who follows up cures of drinking men will see that it is not the way to cure delerium tremens. And the same thing is true of pneumonia patients. It is much more successful to give the patient large quantities of stimulating drugs like strychnia or mineral acids. One of the most useful things for that purpose is red pepper. A patient in that condition can easily take a teaspoon of red pepper in hot soup, and with a great deal of benefit. It acts as a severe local irritant.

Dock did not give his pneumonia patients red pepper, but he did give strychnine. He wrote in 1904: "I cannot yet admit its uselessness in circulatory weakness." A little girl with pneumonia was almost completely comatose. Her hands and feet were cyanotic, her heart weak, her pulse 180. Dock prescribed an increased dose of strychnine because most doctors did not give enough: 1/60 grain every four hours. The girl's tendons had been twitching for the last day and night.

Dock concluded:

> So I would beg you to remember this point as an example of what can be done without any great array of treatment. Now some of you are saying that is all very well in a University Hospital be-

cause nobody cares whether a patient gets any medicine or not and if he does it does not matter because we are impervious to things of that kind, but for the country doctor and cross roads doctor and even the village doctor that sort of treatment will not do. I know a great many cross roads doctors who do just as we do here, where they get only ice bags and the people are satisfied and even begin the treatment themselves.

The ice bag relieves pain.

As regards the ice bag, let me say that you will find always a good deal of objection to using an ice bag in a town where the people have not been broken in. There you will have trouble, but in such a place take a patient who has a great deal of pain, dyspnoea, cough; get your ice bag and put it on before you give your hypodermic and tell them if the patient does not within five or ten minutes quickly show improvement in all these symptoms then you will go ahead and give your hypodermic, but I think in that short time the patient will say he is relieved. The fact that it relieves the pain might be supposed to indicate that it really affects the nerves that are affected; but there is a good deal of doubt as to whether the ice bag can reduce the cold beneath the skin. One can find it out by putting a thermometer into a fissure and putting an ice bag over it. The ice bag lessens the pain and then lessens the frequency of respiration and that it lessens the cough I have not any doubt in the world because I have seen it follow so often that I think the relation is very clear, but if someone tells me if comes from suggestion I don't care.

Empyema

Dock aspirated pus from the chest of many patients who had had pneumonia. When he prepared to tap he said:

One should never put such things in carbolic solution; in fact we have some written rules about that but they have been here so long they are looked on as back numbers. (To nurse): You made it fresh? That is a good thing, because old carbolic solution is almost as full of germs as a cancerous stomach. . . . [The patients] may not have pus in them at first; but they have purulent infection there, and if you are not careful—and up to 1885 nobody was careful —you can't tell whether the presence of pus there came from the operation or the original infection.

Sometimes the puncture was a failure. Once Dock broke the only needle he had. On another occasion he got only "gristly tissue." When he abandoned the attempt, a large subcutaneous hematoma formed. "These little accidents that sometimes happen are alarming."

When Dock obtained thick, creamy pus characteristic of pneumococcal empyema, he recommended drainage by incision. That treatment was not always successful, for one patient returned after three months with continued drainage. The opening had been too small, only one-eighth of an inch. It must be enlarged and a bigger drainage tube inserted.

In 1905 Dock had his students observe a scar with even margins on a patient's chest, the result of an operation four years earlier for abscess of the lung. During the operation some chisling had been done to resect bone. Now there was a swelling at the site of the scar. Dock got grayish white fluid when he aspirated.

DOCK: Does it look like empyematous pus? It looks like pus from where?

STUDENT: From some suppurating joint.

DOCK: It looks more like the pus that comes from necrotic bone, it has a dirty grayish appearance, somewhat watery; so primarily the trouble is necrosis of the bone, a process that sometimes follows empyemic disease. It is not due to any error in the operation, but simply one of the inevitable results of operating on bone.

Counterirritation in Pleurisy

Dock said there is no treatment for pleurisy, but its pain can be controlled by counterirritation. On November 30, 1906, he removed the bandages from a patient whose pleurisy with effusion had been treated by cauterization. He asked a student what he saw.

STUDENT: They might be from a blister, couldn't they?

DOCK: But from the shape and size and position and number it would seem most likely they were done by some sort of cautery.

PATIENT: That is what they are.

DOCK: When were you burnt?

PATIENT: Yesterday.

DOCK: Has it relieved the pain? How bad was it before? What kind of an end was there?

PATIENT: A little narrow end with a button on it.

DOCK (to students): Usually we don't need so many points; usually we use the button end which is about as big as a dime, and a button like that makes a fairly good sized mark, and if there is pain extending from there to there it would be enough to put about three points; e.g., where we treat the sciatic we put the points about four or five inches apart over the thigh. It takes a little experience and practice to tell just how the cautery burn is going to come out. When you put it on the patient doesn't feel it as much as you do yourself. Let's ask him.

PATIENT: I felt it all right.

DOCK: If at the proper temperature the pain is not ever so much as one would expect; but as you are holding the cautery and seeing the thing and smelling the burning flesh, which to me is the most disagreeable part of it, you immediately begin to pull the cautery away and the result is the patient gets a superficial burn that doesn't go through the epidermis, and the next day it is nearly healed. If you burn a little longer then you get a deep burn. It doesn't do any harm and the counter irritation that goes on in the healing has a very beneficial effect.

Some patients bore the scars of cupping, but Dock no longer used that treatment. There was a set of cupping glasses in the hospital if they could be found. Dock said:

They are usually worked by holding a sponge soaked with alcohol and igniting it down in the bottom of the cup; then turning the bottom upward, taking the sponge out and putting the glass over the spot of the body where you want it to work. You can get six or eight cups on; but you must be careful not to get the edge of the glass hot; I have seen some very bad burns produced by nervous operators dropping the glass and giving the patient an ugly burn that would be come infected.

Then Dock showed the students how to put on a dressing: two layers of gauze and nothing else.

Fluid in the Thorax

A student diagnosed encapsulated pleural effusion at the right apex, and Dock differentiated between such an effusion and hydrothorax.

DOCK: Why do you think it is encapsulated?

STUDENT: The pleura would be adherent, so that the fluid would not be able to move around.

DOCK: What is your idea of the movability of pleural fluid in general?

STUDENT: That it would change with the change of position in about half an hour.

DOCK: Why does it not move more rapidly?

STUDENT: The surrounding fluid is more or less adherent.

DOCK: That is quite right. It is an important fact that we don't usually find the fluid in acute pleurisy, or one that was acute in the beginning, as freely movable as from hydrothorax, but it is not necessary to have fibrous adhesions to do that; it is quite enough if the fluid is sticky.

Inflammatory fluid contains albuminous bodies, Dock said, and "[t]hus inflammatory fluid has a higher specific gravity than non inflammatory fluid; the dividing line is 1015; above that it is inflammatory; below that non inflammatory; and the farther we get away from the margin the less inflammatory it is; so 1008 is positively not inflammatory, and 1022 is almost invariably inflammatory."

After 1903 Dock regularly used X rays to help in the diagnosis of pleural effusion. He called

> attention to the skiagraph curve. The right side is clear; the curve of the diaphragm is over the liver and there is an unusual shadow to the right of the middle line, not only to the left of the heart but above that. It looks as if the heart and great vessels were pushed too far to the right or there was something else producing the shadow; and you notice on the left side something that absorbs light from the third rib down, really from the second interspace down, and reaching the stomach area here.

Sometimes he compared skiagraphs taken before and after removal of fluid.

Dock said little about the causes of pleural effusion or hydrothorax. In the case of a woman who three days before had an extensive gynecological operation, he said: "The explanation that we give is that the patient has taken up through the diaphragm through the lymphatic openings, septic material from the abdomen, that is, germs from the seat of operation. The trouble is that when you make a statement of that kind you nearly always call down upon the operator the charge of having had an infected field of operation." The field may not have been infected, but there are many germs in the abdominal cavity anyway. At another time Dock blamed an extensive hydrothorax upon mitral stenosis that dammed back blood in the lungs.

Salt-Free Diet

Fluid of pleural effusion can be removed medically by giving the patient Epsom or Glauber's salts dissolved in as little water as possible. It is "a very disagreeable drink." Dock preferred to cause diuresis with salicylic acid or its salts.[3] They act promptly; they are harmless; and they may have some effect upon the pathological process causing the effusion. However, diuretics do not always work. "You can increase diuresis three or four hundred per cent, but that does not affect the osmotic conditions of the fluid, and it remains as before."

On October 25, 1904, Dock demonstrated a woman with hydrothorax, and as he aspirated her chest she complained:

I can't stand that.

DOCK: You are standing it all right.

PATIENT: Why don't you give me chloroform? Don't stir me up.

DOCK: It would be better for you if you were stirred up a bit.

The woman also complained about the hospital food; it had lost its savor. Dock said that was because her food was prepared without salt. He continued:

> There are also some other points to think about in this connection; that is, changing the absorption of fluid in the body by altering the osmotic pressure of the fluid. Work is being done showing the relation of the reduction of salt in these cases. It is a fact that water stays in because sodium chloride stays in the tissues and keeps water there; so if you can make the sodium chloride less then you relieve the patient, and you do that by putting the patient on sodium chloride starvation, and then the sodium is likely to go down. This works better in pure kidney cases than in heart cases but they use it in heart cases too sometimes.

Dock did not say who "they" were, but a half hour's detective work in the medical library identified one as Fernand Widal and another as Charles Achard. Each had published long papers and many short ones in the 1903 volume of a French journal.[4] The point of all the papers was that sodium chloride retention inevitably results in water retention. Widal and his collaborator had demonstrated this by giving patients with Bright's disease 10 grams of sodium chloride a day for ten days. The result on successive days was

> OEdème pulmonaire. OEdème du scrotum.
>
> Gros oedème des jambes.
>
> Crises épileptiformes. Tous les oedème augmentés.

Three days after sodium chloride was discontinued:

> OEdème diminuent surtout au scrotum et au dos, persiste à la face.

The long paper by Achard in the Taubman Medical Library is marked with pencil in the margin in Dock's habitual manner, and it gives the explanation: "Aujourd'hui leur explication est devenue facile, grâce à la notion d'un méchanisme régulateur qui répartit dans l'ensemble de l'organisme les chlorures retenus et déverse en même temps dans les tissus l'eau necessaire à leur dilution."

Technique of Tapping the Chest

Dock used a patient with pleural effusion following pneumonia to demonstrate the technique of removing fluid from the chest.

> DOCK: There are two reasons in this case for operating. First, to find out whether there is actual fluid there, because if she has interstitial pneumonia it would be proper to hasten resolution, and if she has fluid it would be proper to take it away. If there is pleurisy just from pneumonia, it may go away by itself, but you can never be sure that it will. So we will explore in what is the point of election in such cases, generally in the axilla in the 6th or 7th interspace.
>
> (TO PATIENT). Now this isn't going to hurt you very much.
>
> (TO STUDENTS): An explorative operation in this way is very important. You only explore where you think you are going to get something. For your instrument, you want something that will work well. Don't use a hypodermic needle. About the best thing I know of for exploratory tapping is a machine like this which has a barrel that will take 15 or 20 c.c. and is easily sterilized. It cost $2.50. I had this made to order and they work pretty well. The ordinary needle, if it is long enough, is too heavy. Such an operation requires very little preparation. The danger of infecting the pleura is practically nothing at all provided the needle is sterilized, and you sterilize it by boiling. The skin should be clean, but it is not necessary to go through any complicated process. The next point is that it should never be done in a hurry. As in all operations, you want to put the needle in steadily and slowly, you don't want to show wonderful dexterity with the needle, the way that old

women used to handling a needle could do. We want to fix the interspace with the fingers. I find the wisest way is to take two fingers and put the needle between them or, knowing the general direction, to put down one finger and then get the needle opposite the end of the finger. Beginners usually go too rapidly because they think it will give the patient less pain, and partly on account of a very natural nervousness and disposition to get there as quickly as possible.

(TO PATIENT): It didn't hurt very much, did it?

PATIENT: No sir.

(TO STUDENTS). Most patients will tell you that it doesn't hurt very much. Now, you notice that I took plenty of time to do this. You can't emphasize too often the danger of doing this work in a hurry. You try to make out what the point is passing through. In the skin there is resistance; in the muscle much less resistance. Along the pleura you go into a hollow cavity or else you go into the lung; you can feel the lung tissue in a characteristic way. It feels like a very rotten sponge. When you get into a hollow place you feel it, and then you begin to aspirate and you do it slowly so as to avoid accident.

Then Dock replaced the needle with a cannula and trocar:

I may say for the benefit of those who may have to do this operation in private practice that it is not necessary to have such a large corps of assistants as we are having here. You may have to do it by yourself, with the farmer's wife to hand the basin. You simply have all your instruments lying together; wash him yourself, freeze with a drop of ethyl chloride and pick up your knife; then make your cut in the same breath that you take up the knife with, in a much shorter time than it takes me to tell about it; lay your knife down carefully so as not to hurt it; then get your trocar; and then you pass it slowly after you have the skin cut; have the trocar and cannula fit well, and they will go in almost as they should, and after you find that you are in, then adjust your tube and do the rest. Now we will use today in order to keep our hand in an aspirator; but ordinarily you do this without an aspirator because it costs more than it is worth. They never work, at least if this one works it will be the first one I ever saw; you can get as much aspiration by having a long tube full of boiled water, and having that hang down over the bed. Notice the patient is coughing. That is a symptom that the lung is being touched there by the end of the trocar, or it is expanding and the cough comes from the irritation of the bronchi in the expanding part.

Dock said you should not remove too much fluid at one time. Some doctors boast that they have removed 4,000 cc, but the risk of massive tapping is syncope that will be quick and incurable. When he did remove "about 2,000 c.c." from an elderly man whose arteries were "not what they used to be," the blood pressure fell from 210 to 150. Dock said: "The thing to do was to keep him quiet until it was certain the lung had expanded and was back where it ought to be because if he suddenly developed a twist in the aorta he might not have anything else to bother him, and that within a short time." If only part of the fluid is removed, dyspnea is relieved and the circulation improved. That favors reabsorption of the remaining fluid.

Dock did not approve of tightly binding the good side of the chest in order to make the patient use the side from which fluid had been removed. Instead:

A very useful way to accomplish over action on the right [the diseased] side is to let the patient lean over the arm of an arm chair, taking hold of the lower round, and then practicing deep breathing. The left side will be hampered and the right side will have a chance to extend downward toward the diaphragm and also laterally.

Or

In addition it is useful to have the patient breathing against an obstruction and that can be done with blowing bottles. You have to have them made for your patients after you get out. You have a pair of bottles connected in this way with a blowing tube going in only a short distance, and then another tube beginning at the bottom of one bottle and leading through a system of tubes into the top of another one. The first bottle is filled with water. The patient is taught to blow in that and must be taught to take a deep breath and then force that as steadily and strongly as possible against the pressure of the water into the other bottle.

Some patients blow with their cheeks, and that must be discouraged.

KIDNEY TROUBLE

5.

DOCK READ THE HISTORY OF A MAN
with arteriosclerosis whom he had seen ten years before. Now the man
had come to the University Hospital with headache, failing vision, and
systolic blood pressure "about in the neighborhood of 240 instead of say
140." The student responsible for the patient on the wards said the
twenty-four-hour urine volume had been 2,000 cc. Its specific gravity
was 1,012; albumin was present at 1/5 volume; and there was a moderate number of hyaline and granular casts.

These findings were confusing, and Dock tried unsuccessfully to
differentiate between interstitial and parenchymatous nephritis. He
could not decide whether the patient's kidneys would be found to be
small and pale, small and mottled, or small and red. He said. "But of
course there may be areas in the kidney that show a good deal of parenchymatous change and parts that show tubular change, so examination
of a part of the kidney may be just as misleading as an examination of
the urine." Dock did not explain the characteristics of the two forms of
kidney disease. They were clearly laid out in Osler's textbook[1] and
Dock expected the students to know them. Their answers to his questions showed that they did.

Examining the Urine: Volume

Twenty-four-hour urine collection was routine on Dock's service in the
University Hospital, and he urged his students to continue the practice
after they graduated. He said:

> Generally one does not want to be carrying a 24 hours' sample off
> to one's office, so an easy way is to get the patient a big wide-

89

UNIVERSITY HOSPITAL

DEPARTMENT OF INTERNAL MEDICINE

URINE EXAMINATION

Name ....Date....................

In-patient, No................Out-patient, No.................

Extra-........Dr. ....Diagnosis ....

......Sample, hour......24 hours......voided......catheter......

Quantity ....Specific Gravity ......Reaction......Color......

Clear ....Turbid ....Floaters....................

Albumin: Heat and nitric acid................................

" Acetic and ferrocyanide.............................

" Heller's ....

Albumose: method ....

Glucose ....Fehling......quantity........................

K O H...............phenylhydracin..................

fermentation ....quantity......... ....

Bile-coloring ....foam.........Gmelin...............

Urobilin .... Indican......................

Acetone .... Diacetic acid................

Ferric-chloride reaction .... Diazo......................

Sediment, amount ....color.........appearance..........

Microscopic: crystals ....

red blood cells, No.............; condition...................

leukocytes No. ....; kind.......................

epithelial cells ....; kind....................

Casts ....

....

......................cylindroids ....

Spermatozoa ....Bacteria ....

....

Protozoa ....

Remarks ....

....

....

....

....

Examined by...........................

FIGURE 8. Form used in Dock's department for reporting urinalyses.

mouthed bottle marked with a [blank] of any kind of paint or ink, so that the patient can easily read off what the total quantity is. The best way is to have it marked with c.c.'s. Anybody can read those off and make a note what the quantity is. Then you have 24 hours safe and measured. That is done at the house. You can even have the Sp. G. taken at home. If you furnish the people with a urinometer and show any, half-way intelligent person how to use it there is usually somebody in the house who can do it to satisfaction.

If the patient is a pregnant woman or has diabetes,

you want samples for daily examination, and you get those by giving bottles every morning, large enough for your purpose, 6 or 8 ounces, and that sample should represent the whole 24 hours, and it should be sterile and kept in such a way that the urine will not decompose, and you will find it much easier to have the thing done in the meanest private home than in a large hospital. You can have the bottle boiled and having taken the same amount of care with a urine bottle as with a milk bottle—and that is little enough, as everybody knows.

Examining the Urine: Albumin

The student had said that albumin was 1/5 in volume. James Rae Arneill,[2] Dock's first assistant until 1903, described the meaning of that term in his book, Clinical Diagnosis and Urinalysis:

A test-tube partially filled with perfectly clear urine is heated to boiling over a flame. A cloudiness may result, due to albumin or earthy phosphates. A little nitric acid is then added; if the cloudiness is due to phosphates, the urine immediately becomes clear, while if it is due to albumin it remains or may even increase. . . . An idea of the amount of albumin may be obtained by observing . . . the bulk of the precipitated albumin, 1/10, 1/4, 1/2, etc., will give the approximate quantity.[3]

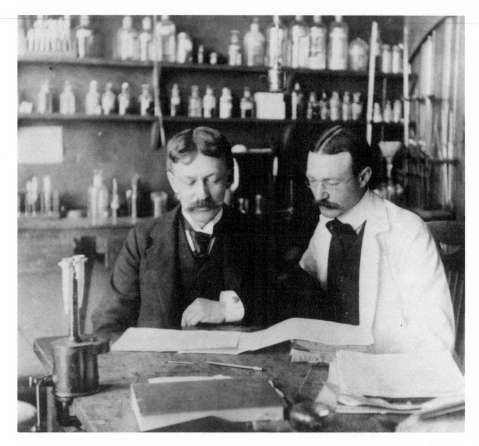

FIGURE 9. George Dock and James Arneill in Dock's office-laboratory. (From Michigan Historical Collections, Bentley Historical Library)

Dock said he was always sorry when he saw "people working in a country where they haven't gas. The meanest thing to boil urine with is an alcohol lamp." It is important to use nitric acid rather than acetic, for acetic precipitates mucus as well as albumin. He thought the size of flakes precipitated has diagnostic importance: large flakes nearly always indicate kidney disease.

During a long discussion of a patient with nephritis, Dock said:

Now he tells us in the history that he at one time had 80% albumin. What do you think of that?

STUDENT: It must be a mistake.

DOCK: He made a very great mistake of expressing the quantity of albumin by bulk in decimal figures. What the doctor did, no doubt, was this,—he precipitated the albumin. He probably found the tube with 4/5 urine; he put this into percentages. How much albumin can a man have? 3% is very large—1% will give a great deal more than 4/5 volume; he probably had 1/2%. When we look at the tube containing albumin it is common to say it contains 1/4, or 3/4 or whatever it is, but when we have weighed the dry albumin or we have used some other measure that may be more exact, then we may put the results in percentages; otherwise we can lead only to misunderstanding.

Once a patient with kyphosis and a fractured rib said he got round-shouldered milking cows. Dock said: "This is a disease of the bones that goes along with stiffening of the bones, and you frequently get albuminose in the urine. We will examine for albuminose by the cold nitric acid test, which dissolves on heating and then comes down again on cooling." Dock did not discuss the bone disease further or the peculiar albumose in the urine.[4]

Examining the Urine: Collecting Sediment

Dock passed around a specimen of urine.

DOCK: What do you think about that?

STUDENT: It is light colored and very slightly cloudy.

DOCK: You might think it is clear, yet when you look at it carefully, either it is not clear or else it is in a very dirty glass, and that is not unlikely where the water is so hard.

A few threadlike bodies were called floaters. They were made up of pus cells, mucus, epithelial cells and germs of various kinds. Dock said that "They come from deep in the urethra, possibly in the curve of the urethra, and they always indicate local inflammation there, the cause of which we cannot tell." And there may be "clap threads." "[I]f you hold the urine up to the light it looks muddy—when you find that kind of thing, I think you are warranted in making a fatal prognosis."

Dock described Osler's method of collecting sediment: "If you are carrying bottles home, carry them upside-down tightly stoppered, and by the time you get home you have a sediment on the stopper; then carefully turn the bottle right side up, without shaking, and taking the stopper carefully, smear over the slide and there you have your sediment, a sediment showing casts, cells, etc."

Other methods are described as well by Dock:

> Lots of people have an idea that to get a sediment you must let the urine stand for any unknown number of hours. If you want to get it quickly a centrifuge is the thing; so that very profitable apparatus —you cannot get a more useful instrument for from $9 to $15— will save more time than [blank], especially if you make the precipitation before the patient,—it has a very marvellous effect, the whirling arm of the centrifuge has highly hypnotic powers. One could hardly get along in general practice without obstetric forceps but the centrifuge is more important. You can borrow the forceps from your neighbor, the need occurs only once in a while.

There was the problem of getting the sediment onto a slide:

> There are all sorts of ways of getting the stuff out of the centrifuge tube. I have seen a doctor whirl urine in an electric centrifuge machine ten minutes, then take the tube upside-down over a sink and let out most of the urine and then let a few drops run out on a slide. Such recklessness is likely to wash out everything.

Dock described "the Boston pipette method; not because it came from Boston but was originated by a man of that name, Dr. Napoleon Boston." Another name is "the lazy interne's method." However,

> This must be done with brains like everything else. The handiest way is to have a pipette that will reach just about to the bottom of the centrifuge tube; the tube should not be too narrow for another reason. If it is only two or three millimeters [it] has a high capillarity, and perhaps the very part of the stuff you want you can't

get unless you blow through it; so the best way is to have a long straight tube, perfectly round at both ends, and put it down to the bottom of the centrifuge tube and let the stuff carefully run up by letting the air out through your finger. Then you will have all the sediment in 5 or 6 or 7 or 8 c.c. of urine. It is important to wipe the outside of the tube first; if you do not, then the first of the drops you put on the glass slide will be pure urine from the upper part. You want a large drop, a slide 4 × 5 or any length of glass of that kind, and then you get a series of large drops lying side by side, and then you are quite certain you have on your slide every bit of sediment in the urine. Each drop should be large and high and it is easy to make it high if the glass is clean.

Don't let the drop dry, for then the sediment will be covered with salts; draw off the water by touching the edge of the drop with filter paper. Stain with ordinary basic dyes but always with tuberculin stain. Dock's junior colleague David Murray Cowie had found that bacilli in smegma stain like tubercle bacilli, and he had shown how to tell the difference.[5]

Every doctor should have a microscope in his office, and there was always one available in the clinic. Dock suggested:

What one should do with casts of that kind would be to get a cover glass over that same drop, center the same casts with low power, and bring down the high power and find whether it is a blood cast or not. . . . Why do you put the diaphragm on? I think it safe to say that about 9/10 of the casts in practice are not seen when they look for them because they do not arrange the diaphragm properly.

Once a student saw a highly refractile cast.

DOCK: What is there about it?

STUDENT: It looks segmented. I do not know what would give it that appearance.

DOCK: What do you think it is, Detweiler?

DETWEILER: I think it is wool, some kind of hair.

Dock used no other tests of kidney function, "But we hear and read a great deal about testing the renal functions with various chemicals. As a matter of fact none of those methods are superior to the old and some-what rough and ready methods of testing." The phenolsulphonphtha-lein test was not described until two years after Dock left Ann Arbor.[6]

Bacturia and Hematuria

A patient with pus in his urine had not had a rectal examination. Dock said, "I remember now how it was that it hadn't been done. He was to have been examined in the G.U. clinic; but even if you are not a G.U. specialist you should examine the prostate." The urological surgeons in the University Hospital removed stones and tuberculous kidneys, but Dock often had to make the initial diagnosis. Once a patient with mild diabetes, a history of stone, and streaks of red in his urine was referred to Dock because the surgeons had failed in an attempted cystoscopy. Dock remarked: "You never pass a sound at once in such a man. You ex-amine the urine first, for you might have to pass an instrument on a man who has sepsis the next hour, who may have severe symptoms, and it would be hard to make him think it was not your manipulations that made him have symptoms, and, in fact, he might be right."

When there were many leucocytes in the urine, Dock had to deter-mine the site of suppuration, and if a kidney were tuberculous, which one.

The further examination shows this: if we let him pass his urine in two parts the last part contains just the same kind of pus that the first part does so that evidently the pus comes from above the ure-thra altogether. There are two things that can be done, however: first, it would be a good thing, if we had the proper apparatus, to cystoscope the patient and see if the pus comes from one or both kidneys. However cystoscopes and instruments for getting the urine from either kidney are not altogether easy for a fresh physi-cian to use, but I would strongly urge you, if there is a chance, to cultivate this instrument. But we can get at it this way. If you mas-sage a kidney you get things out that otherwise would not come, you can get blood and epithelial cells and some casts shortly after-ward. Acting on that fact people have massaged the kidneys separatey in order to see if they could get a change in the urine after each. . . . You might suppose the urine coming from the other kidney would make the results difficult to interpret, but they don't.

When there was pus in the urine Dock prescribed urotropin, hexamethylamine that breaks down in the urine into formaldehyde. Cushny said it was a superior urinary antiseptic. Salicylic acid and carbolic acid are no good; they are excreted in an inactive form. If all else fails, use boracic acid. However, in every instance the infection must be considered tuberculous until numerous examinations show this is not the case. A diagnosis of tuberculosis might be confirmed by the tuberculin test, but in 1901 Dock said the tuberculin they were supplied was unreliable. A suspension of urinary sediment might be injected into a guinea pig, and in at least one instance of doubtful diagnosis the guinea pig died of unmistakable tuberculosis within a month.

A patient had been passing bloody urine for a month. Dock said the first thing to think about was tuberculosis, but the tuberculin test was negative. A new growth might occur at any time of life, and Dock favored that diagnosis on account of the duration of hemorrhage. Treatment was purely empirical. "The pharmacologists tell us it is no good. The drug we use is acetate of lead, one to three grains three times a day. This can be given for a couple of weeks with great advantage. If the hemorrhage is not controlled in a short time, the drug should be stopped." In this case, bleeding did stop, so the urine could be examined. It contained large cells like those from a new growth, but the urine passed in the middle of the morning contained spermatozoa. Was this blood from the seminal vesicles, for sometimes very alarming bloody emissions follow gonorrhea? According to Dock: "An emission could be ruled out. In such cases you will tell the patient quite plainly what you want to know. The patient denies another cause, but you know how careful you have to be about believing some statements."

A student, seeing fluid come from a urinary fistula, called it an exudate.

DOCK: What are exudates? That is sophomore work. Give me the best definition you can.

STUDENT: I know, but I can't tell.

DOCK: If you understand you can tell; if you can't tell, I don't believe you understand.

STUDENT. It is fluid covering two tissues.

DOCK: That is what you might give if you had only studied Latin and not medicine, but this is medicine. Hincks?

STUDENT: I think it must come from the blood.

DOCK: Great Scott! Howe? Hunt?

STUDENT: It is fluid coming from lymph and collecting in a small mass.

DOCK: Jickling?

STUDENT: I think it is fluid excreted from any part of the body on a free surface.

DOCK: Well, that would apply to urine, wouldn't it?

STUDENT: On a serous surface.

DOCK: Well, how about diphtheria? Could you call that an exudate?

STUDENT: On a mucous surface.

DOCK: Then you have enlarged your definition, didn't you? Gregory?

STUDENT: An effusion upon a free surface.

DOCK: I will expect the whole class to be able to hand in a written definition of an exudate at the next clinic. I remember a striking example of that I heard in Virchow's [clinic]. He was talking about the development of bacterial diagnosis, which was always a thorn in his side, and on being asked what a serum was, said "Anything that isn't exact urine."

Palpation of the Kidney

Dock asked:

Never felt a kidney before? That is too bad. In order to feel a kidney, if it is difficult to feel, you have to take some pains; if it is easy to feel, you can't make a mistake. Have the patient lying down and get your left hand—the right kidney is the one we are most likely to feel—under the 11th and 12th ribs, and press up quite firmly, and then you get the other hand just below the ribs in this position, and get the patient to take a deep breath, just as deep as he can, and keep your finger tips a little bit down, and usually you feel the kidney coming down under your fingers; but if you don't feel it coming down, then you shove your fingers in very briskly so as to meet the other hand, and then when the patient takes an inspiration you feel the kidney slipping back. . . . You will recognize it by its peculiar slippery feeling. If you get it between your fingers, the patient nearly always says that it causes soreness. The pain people feel when you squeeze the kidney varies a great deal, some describe it as a feeling of nausea, others don't seem to have very much pain from it.

Palpation might reveal nephroptosis or floating kidney, common conditions at that time. Once when Dock discovered a floating kidney and a dropped stomach, he said: "It is quite likely when she is standing the kidney drags on the pyloric end of the stomach."

Retention

When he examined a man with elevated brown and red spots, unequal pupils, gastric crises, loss of patellar reflexes and slight incoordination, Dock found in the middle of the abdomen a long oval mass as big as a fetal head. He was sure it had not been there in the morning. A student said the patient might have a full bladder. The patient was sent out to urinate, but when he returned the mass was not much smaller.

DOCK: Let's get a catheter, bring him in here and let Walsh catheterize him as a reward of virtue. How would you do it in practice?

STUDENT: I would wash my hands and sterilize with bichloride and boil the catheter and put a little lubricant over it.

DOCK: It is really very simple; you have everything ready; and it is not a bad way to have the patient do the preliminary washing himself, and you have solutions and cotton and keep a hand at the site of operation all the time. You don't need much lubricant on the catheter; just enough to get the end started. It is just like a stomach tube; after it makes a start there is no trouble getting it down.

They got over a liter of urine. Dock prescribed strychnine for atony of the bladder and sent the patient to the neurology clinic.

Dock admonished the class:

Please notice the pains that we took to avoid infecting the bladder. It is always very proper to do so, but always interesting to hear, too, of the risks people will run safely. . . . I wanted to examine his urine so I asked somebody to get a sterilized catheter, but he said, "I have it with me," and he pulled it out of his pocket. I said it was unsafe to use without sterilizing, but he said that was no use; for sixteen years he had never passed water in any other way and he had never any trouble at all. So I told him to pass it his own way. So he lubricated the catheter with saliva, and the urine came out perfectly clear.

Things were different when Dock was a student: "A man who is now one of the leading surgeons in the United States showed me in my undergraduate days a good way to carry a catheter; he cut a hole in the sweat band of his hat and put the catheter inside with the outer end through the hole. Fortunately the days of asepsis dawned before I got outside, and I never carried mine that way."

Not all retention is pathological. Dock said: "Holding the urine is one of the commonest causes of irritation of the bladder and other diseases. School teachers are notoriously subject to bladder disease which is usually attributed to the necessity of holding their urine for long periods." At another time Dock brought a newborn girl to the clinic. She had not yet passed water. The bowels had moved, so there was probably no malformation. Could there be a uric acid infarct? He said the best treatment is a hot water bottle over the genitals. At the bottom of the transcript Dock wrote in pencil: "This done—water passed one hour later."

Uremia

A paraplegic child, injured by gunshot, had been in the hospital a long time. Dock described her present condition:

> Following almost complete cessation of urine secretion, she gets the symptoms I have described,—the tendency to vomiting, nausea, etc., in a patient without any explanation for it. The tendency to sleep, which gradually passes over to a mild stupor, so that Sunday the patient took little notice of the surroundings and answered very slowly. To say a patient of that kind has apoplexy of the brain is not necessary. The physician should recognize uremia in the early stages and not wait until patient gets severe and unmistakable signs; unmistakable when you know about the case, but puzzling when you see the patient for the first time in that condition.

Treatment requires promptness and is very simple. There are three means to bring about excretion: brisk purgation, sweating induced by hot air or hot water baths, and large doses of diuretin. Dock suggested: "You might put hot applications to the lumbar region to have counter irritating effect on the kidneys. If you used mustard plaster, it would be a slow, painful method." The prognosis is doubtful.

Nephritis

A patient had been sent to the University Hospital when his physician found albumin in his urine, and he had been in the hospital three months before he was presented at an afternoon clinic.

DOCK: What diagnosis do you make?

STUDENT: Bright's disease.

DOCK: What is that?

STUDENT: Inflammation of the kidneys; parenchymatous and interstitial.

DOCK: What is this?

STUDENT: I think it is acute.

DOCK: It began in December and has been running three months. Either it is chronic or else an acute case that has run too long; I don't mean has been allowed to run, but for various reasons has run longer than one should expect. What can you say from the examination of the urine about the case? Does that enable you to say whether it is acute, chronic, or what?

STUDENT: I would say chronic.

DOCK: Why?

STUDENT: On account of the small amount and high specific gravity.

DOCK: How small is the amount?

STUDENT. One day he passed 100 c.c.; another day, 300 c.c.

DOCK (reading): 400 c.c. one day; 600, another; and 600 yesterday. How about the specific gravity?

STUDENT: It is 1018 to 1025. It is not interstitial.

DOCK: Why?

STUDENT: On account of the high specific gravity and because casts are not abundant.

DOCK: But if he has only 600 in 1018, that wouldn't be high, would it? You have to divide the solid contents by the quantity. That means that the specific gravity would be really low.

While Dock and the student were discussing the patient, other students had been preparing slides of the urinary sediment.

DOCK: What are our friends finding?

STUDENT: Most of the cells don't seem round cells. They look very much like leukocytes, and other cells have irregular shapes that look as if they might come from lower layers of epithelial cells of mucous membrane. There are hyalin and epithelial cells and one granular cast.

DOCK: Suppose you draw a picture of them on the blackboard.

The picture the student drew is copied in the transcript, and the next three-and-one-half pages are used to record the dialog between Dock and students on the nature of casts: epithelial casts, granular casts, glossy red hyalin casts, and pale waxy casts. One cast had "a very definite shape." Dock remarked:

Not to prolong your misery too much, it seems to me it is a spiral. You might suppose it got spiral from coming down through the convoluted tubules; but it would be hard to explain how it could get down through the straight tubules, so it isn't supposed that these casts are formed in the convoluted tubules; but formed simply on account of their growing through the apices where they take their shape. Their shape may be explained as analogous to a cook making figures on icing. She makes them by letting the icing run out of a cone; so when fluid runs through a small opening it has a tendency to take a spiral form. That cast has no diagnostic importance to justify all the time I have been speaking about it.

Dock said the sediment must be stained for tubercle bacilli.

Suppose we fail to find evidence of TBc and come to the conclusion that the patient has acute or chronic parenchymatous nephritis, what would you do?

STUDENT. I think the indications are to relieve the kidneys as much as possible, put the patient to bed and at rest; give him a light liquid diet and allow him to have what water he wants.

DOCK: Can that be carried too far?

STUDENT: Yes.

DOCK: Yes, it is very easy. I remember a patient with a similar condition of the urine, who was advised to drink all the water possible and he took twelve quarts of water a day, which is too much for anybody to drink.

The patient's red cell count was 4,850,000, the white cell count 6,621, and the hemoglobin 90%. Dock thought that the patient should have a red cell count of 6,000,000 and that the "blood formation is below normal." Iron might irritate his kidneys, and in such a case where the patient cannot take it . . . and really needs iron, and experience shows that the thing is a very good thing to furnish, you have to give it in another way, in their water, in the yolk of egg and in green vegetables. So we will keep the patient in bed for a short time; give him for diet a certain amount of meat, a good deal of milk and egg including the yolk of egg. We will let him have red meat once a day, three or four eggs a day, along with vegetables of various kinds and milk.

When a student said he would "cut out meat diet at first," Dock replied:

The idea was a meat diet containing extractive matter would irritate the kidney and in that way keep up irritation; and there were curious developments of that,—take white meat, like breast of chicken; that did not have as much extractive matter in it as red meat did. But it has been shown very clearly that white meat is practically the same as red meat . . . so far as the kidneys are concerned. How about salt?

STUDENT. It might be eliminated.

DOCK: What is the idea of eliminating it?

STUDENT: It causes increased irritation.

DOCK: That is the theory. It is very interesting and one the young doctor should make himself posted about by reading and one on which he can make useful observations. . . . A good way to do is to give him bread without salt and butter without salt. It is usually prepared by washing the butter, but the salt can be taken out and the taste for unsalted butter is very easily acquired. On the continent of Europe nobody eats it; it is about as bad to eat salted butter as to eat oleomargarine that they describe in the Jungle[7] in this country. How about medicine?

Dock agreed with Osler that "For the persistent albuminuria . . . we have no remedy of the slightest value."[8] Dock remarked: "We will watch the albumin and casts and see how he does under treatment. If he improves we will let him continue on that diet and let him out, but you have to be careful how you let such a patient out, especially in winter time." As for prognosis:

The financial condition of the patient is of great importance in prognosis of kidney disease. If we could send this patient now to Southern California or Florida or South Carolina, he will undoubtedly have a much better chance of getting well than he has here. It may be an instance of chronic nephritis that may have to be treated for many years. In such a case one would examine the eye grounds. That has been done and found negative. As it has been running along for three months one should expect chronic nephritis that would show itself in the eye grounds and blood vessels, and the patient might be one that experience shows always die easily. Here, however, we have no changes in the eye grounds and none in the circulatory organs; so in a way he represents a favorable case. . . . You need to note the signs of uraemia and must be ready to apply the treatment for it.

Nephritis of Pregnancy

On March 27, 1907, Dock brought a patient to the clinic because he wanted to show one with acute parenchymatous nephritis. The woman's face was swollen and discolored, and her urine contained red blood cells, casts, and more than 3/4 albumin. She had been pregnant, but because fetal movements had stopped in the seventh month, her uterus had been emptied. Dock said: "Pregnancy nephritis is characterized by a marked diminution in the amount of urine, high specific gravity, large amounts of albumin and also enormous numbers of casts; we can't get in any other condition except acute scarlatinous nephritis one that shows as many different kinds of casts." Dock said the lesion is in the glomeruli.

The patient had a high systolic blood pressure, over 200 mm Hg. Such patients do not die of uremia but of apoplexy. The treatment for "high tension in the capillaries" is the dose of nitroglycerine recommended by Osler: 10 drops three times a day. Tablets are no good; give nitroglycerine by mouth in a 1% solution. Dock said: "You simply get in on the tongue, and anybody who has doubts about the effects may put ten drops on his tongue and see what happens." Then Dock launched into a long discussion of uremic convulsions:

It is one of the most terrible things you can get ahold of. An apparently healthy woman will be well one day and dead the next. So one should look for what kind of symptoms?

STUDENT: You would tell them to look out for delerium.

DOCK. Yes, but what else?

STUDENT: For signs of shock.

DOCK: You must not tell people to look out for signs of shock, but tell them what signs to look for. If you stand around and look wise you will have everybody terribly rattled and the woman will up and have a convulsion. You ought to tell them to look out for such things as mind wandering or delerium or anything queer about her; if she stops moving her arms or legs or has spasms. You should say, "Don't get alarmed about those things; that is part of the disease. I know exactly what to do; send for me."

But what should he do? Give milk and diuretin to promote diuresis, and give calomel up to 120 grains a day. Bathe the patient in bed with hot water, and give hot drinks to promote sweating.

Dock asked whether meat or milk is bad for the kidneys. Is the albumin in the urine the albumin in the diet?

Now, the question is, what is it in the meat that is bad? Is it the albuminous substances or something else? It has been supposed that it is not the albumin in the meat or any albuminous substance in the meat, but that it is the so-called extractives, the undigestible substances, especially salts of all kinds, organic and inorganic. That is pretty well believed and a proper development of that theory is that salt is one of the most deleterious substances. In fact in the last five years that in nephritis salt in excess is irritating to the kidneys; milk contains little salt so it can be looked on as a salt free diet.

But do not give too much milk; you will flood the tissues and cause edema. Add eggs if you "are not afraid of a little albumin." Give cream, toast, bread, cereals, any kind of plain starchy food, but do not give beef tea. But what should a doctor do if the patient is doing everything she should but still has nephritis?

STUDENT: I think those are the cases where blood-letting is practiced.

DOCK: Why should you bleed her? I don't believe you would practice much if you went around bleeding women that way.

On a follow-up presentation three days later the patient felt well. There was now no edema of the legs, and she "is doing just as post puerperal albuminuria or nephritis ought to do if it is to get well, but is always a thing that may have sudden exacerbations." She was passing larger quantities of urine: 2,600, 2,700, 2,800 cc a day with low specific gravity. Albumin was still present, but Dock attributed that to pus from her gynecological problem. Her headache and dimness of vision, Dock said, were caused by the nitroglycerine, so he substituted amyl nitrite or sodium nitrite to control her blood pressure. Dock asked:

And what other things has she besides that? She was, for example, in a bed in a hospital that notwithstanding disparaging remarks about it, is still in the ring; she had a nurse taking care of her and looking after her; she had you to look after her, she had me; and a number of other people looking after her very carefully and prepared to see when anything dangerous happened, and those are even more important than diuretin and nitroglycerine.

Would the problem recur?

Oh no, that is not necessary at all; that is, a woman may have a severe nephritis, may be so sick that it is necessary to induce premature labor to save life, there may be enormous quantities of albumin and all kinds of casts; yet such an individual not only can get over that but actually can get pregnant and have all the predisposing causes for nephritis and yet not get nephritis. That has a very important bearing sociologically, and is very important for the doctor to know.

Her doctor at home ought to know that she has had acute nephritis. There should be very careful examination of her urine every two or three weeks for the next year and then at decreasing intervals to twice a year as long as she lives.

UNIVERSITY HOSPITAL

DEPARTMENT OF INTERNAL MEDICINE

BLOOD EXAMINATION

Name ....Date ....Hour........

In-patient, No.................Out-patient, No................ ...

Extra ....Dr. ....Diagnosis ....

Fresh drop: Flow........Color.......... Consistence...........

Microscopic: Red cells—Size...........Shape ....

        Color ....relative number..........rolls ....

Leukocytes, number...........other characteristics...............

Plates ....Fibrin ....

Parasites ....

Number of cells, red...............Method....................

Number of cells, white.............Method....................

Hemoglobin ....Method....................

Specific Gravity ....Method....................

Differential count, No....................red cells.............

    small lymphocytes ....microcytes............

    large lymphocytes ....macrocytes...........

    transitional ....poikilocytes...........

    polynuclear ....vacuolated.............

    eosinophile polynuclear ....normoblasts...........

    eosinophile mononuclear ....megaloblasts...........

    myelocytes ....undetermined..........

    mast cells ....

    degenerates ....

....

Other observations ....

....

Remarks ....

....

....

....

             Examined by............................

FIGURE 10. Form used in Dock's department for reporting examinations of the blood.

DISEASES OF THE BLOOD

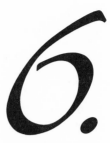

ON JANUARY 23, 1900, DOCK BROUGHT
an anemic woman to the clinic. She had been examined by a student
who reported her red cell count to be 1.6 million and her hemoglobin
concentration to be 25.[1] Dock said the low color index is characteristic
of secondary anemia; the blood-forming organs had been paralyzed by
prolonged anemia. The white count was 4,300. The student did not
report a differential count, but three months before Dock had reprimanded a student for not making one. Dock used the occasion for an
impromptu lecture on examination of the blood.

At that time forty-five members of the class were taking a special
course in examination of the blood, but Dock thought that

> [o]ne would by no means be a master in blood examinations by
> doing this, because there are an enormous number of things that
> can be learned only by practice. Another point is that many people
> have the idea that the whole thing can be learned in the time that
> it would take to read an ordinary book on the subject. It is a very
> great advantage if one can begin the study of the blood with some
> other person who already has gone through that, because there are
> a great many things that can be cleared up better by the assistance
> of another person.

When out in practice, the student should continue to examine every
blood sample he can obtain.

Taking a Sample of Blood

During Dock's time in Ann Arbor, blood was never obtained by venipuncture.[2] Dock usually pricked the end of a finger with a sharp
instrument.

As you probably know a great many people take blood from the ear. I don't think I mentioned this year why I don't do that. I used to stick it more frequently, but it seems to be an awkward place to get at, especially in a woman, the hair gets in the way. Then again it is not easy to get a drop and then have the blood stopped; on the other hand when we want to get a lot of blood then the ear is a very good place. You make a deep cut and an ear will bleed long enough to get 200 covers. . . . In anemic people you sometimes get very little blood [from the finger] and the temptation is always to squeeze on the finger, but never do that under any circumstances.

A sample must be obtained quickly, and

the only way to do it quickly is to have practice. If you have dust, you can't get a good drop. The thing then is to have the finger clean. The best way to do this is to have an ordinary towel wet at one end with either warm or cold water and rub the finger vigorously, especially rubbing along with the papillae of the finger. Then you must get the finger dry. Then you stick it, wipe off the first drop and then take the second drop just as it comes out on either your slide or your cover glass.

Dock preferred slides to cover glasses, for slides are more durable and can be mailed. He said not to prick the finger with a needle, for the round point causes a great deal of pain, "[b]ut better than all else is an instrument modeled after the acne cutter that dermatologists use. It makes a clean cut and heals quickly, and doesn't hurt. The width of the instrument seems to prevent it from causing pain."

To measure coagulation time, Dock suggested two ways:

First, we get a drop of blood under the cover glass on a slide and watch it under the microscope and see when the fibrin forms and by timing it, you will be able to see when the fibrin network begins and when it develops. Second, take a half dozen cover glasses, put a drop of blood on each one, scratch over the blood with a needle and when you begin, you will very easily see there is no fibrin, but, if coagulation begins, you will see you are scratching through a clot. You notice when the clot begins and when it is fully formed.

Make smears on at least six cover glasses or slides, and stain the smears. At that time Dock used hematoxylin and eosin. Once a student failed to stain a smear. Dock snorted that one could make a diagnosis on an unstained smear as well as on a stained one. At the next clinic, Dock apologized to the student; he had seen more on the stained than on the unstained smear.

Estimating Hemoglobin

Dock noted: "If you get into the habit of wiping off the first drop of blood with a towel or filter paper you will notice that not all bloods color the towel or filter paper in the same way. The stain is deeper in some cases than in others. I have long been in the habit of noticing that." Once he complained: "This is a very poor towel, usually old ones are the only kind we have in the clinic."

Dock adopted the Tallqvist method as soon as it was described in the May 1900 issue of the *St. Paul Medical Journal*.[3] Thereafter it was frequently mentioned in the transcript, randomly spelled with one or two *l*'s. On April 30, 1907, it was for the only time spelled with two *l*'s and a *v*.

The color of a drop of blood on a piece of white filter paper is compared with the color of printed spots on a scale graduated in percentages. "With a scale of this kind we have a series of figures varying by tens so that we can get a count that may be five or more degrees off on either side." Dock said the Tallqvist scale would soon be commercially available; in the meantime he purloined the one included in the publication.

Four years later Dock used a Miescher apparatus "that cost $35." It is a cylindrical chamber divided into two compartments set over an aperture in a stage resembling that of a microscope.[4] Blood from a standard pipette, diluted with water, is placed in one compartment, and its color is compared with that of a red glass wedge moved under the other compartment until the depth of colors match. The concetration of hemoglobin is read from a scale attached to the wedge. Tallqvist and Miescher results were always reported in percentage of some unstated normal value, never in grams per 100 cc of blood.

Dock cautioned students against errors. Some persons have bad color sense for red and cannot pick out red yarn from gray. He told of a student who could distinguish cherries from leaves on a tree only by their shape. Students should have their vision tested for they need good color vision to distinguish stained tubercle bacilli as well as for estimating hemoglobin. Dock had had his own vision tested. He also advised students and staff alike to repeat each observation four times, and he compared results obtained with the Tallqvist scale with the "more accurate" Miescher results. Blood from an anemic patient, Dock said,

> flows very poorly., it looks more like wine than blood; and when it gets on the towel it makes a very pale spot there and when it is on the Tallqvist you will see that it reads in the neighborhood of 60, but we also see that on the filter paper the drop is not uniform. Against the light you will see that the paper around the red drop is wet. That is a very important sign, because it indicates that the coloring matter of the blood is not even distributed.

Counting Red Blood Cells

> DOCK STATED: It is difficult to see how one can do satisfactory work without a blood counter and without knowing how to use it. A blood counter costs about $15 or $16. It is unfortunate that these things are so expensive, but they are, and one has to make up his mind either to do that sort of work or go without the apparatus and the work, just as fifty years ago a doctor had to make up his mind whether he would buy a pair of obstetrical forceps or lose a child now and then for want of it.[5] . . . You count with a mechanical stage, although I think one could become so expert by sliding the preparation with the fingers that he could do good work without it.

Counts made by two persons may differ by 100,000.

If a student did not have a hemocytometer, he could get by using the Hammerschlag method of estimating the specific gravity of the blood. The specific gravity of a series of mixtures of chloroform and benzene is determined using a urinometer. A drop of blood either rises or falls in a mixture, and the specific gravity "we know corresponds very closely to the hemoglobin strength." The cell count can then be guessed on the assumption that the cells have a normal color index.

White Cells

White cells were counted using a hemocytometer, but a differential count could be made on a smear. Once Dock reported differential counts on 182 cells and on 1,000 cells. He insisted that at least six smears be made at one time, and he justified this by citing Ehrlich's dictum that megaloblasts could not be declared absent unless one had looked at six smears.

Dock had students examine smears in the clinic, and he told a student to look through a microscope with both eyes open.

DOCK: I will get you to come up and examine these slides. What did you see, Collins?

STUDENT: I just glanced at them.

DOCK: You never ought to glance at a preparation; you always ought to look carefully at it. It is a bad habit. I had rather hear somebody tell me something about it before I proceed to tell what I know about it. Therein lies instruction.

Dock knew Ehrlich's work well, and before Dock left Ann Arbor he had published eight papers on leukemia. Consequently he could not resist the impulse to lecture on cell morphology, and a transcript of a detailed account occupies thirteen pages of transcript. Dock drew pictures on the blackboard, and he told his students to draw what they saw. His published papers contain reproductions of his camera lucida drawings and photomicrographs, but there are many more originals in the rare book room of Michigan's Taubman Medical Library.[6]

Anemia

An emaciated girl had a red cell count of 3,500,000 and a hemoglobin concentration of 30%. Dock said the blood is characteristic of chlorosis, although the girl did not have a dark green color. He referred students to Niemeyer's description of chlorosis,[7] "one of the most common disorders in females between the ages of 14 and 20." The girl was constipated, but Dock did not believe constipation causes chlorosis. Cancer of the stomach could be ruled out, because of her age and because no lactic acid was in her gastric contents. She should use cold baths, go out of doors and take exercise. The specific treatment is inorganic iron in the form of Blaud's pills.[8] At present, Dock said, there is the general idea that inorganic iron is ineffective, "yet we have more testimony to the value of inorganic iron that to any other drug except quinine."

Anemia follows blood loss, and whenever you see a patient who is pale, examine the stool for blood. The patient was put on a hemoglobin-free diet when that was done. Dock said many persons have hemorrhages every day but do not know it. "The patient says he fainted at stool but there is no blood, and you go there and see there is blood." Here again, treatment is inorganic iron. Iron in many forms, iron filings and rust, has been successfully used, but Blaud's pills are the most convenient. They should be freshly made. Dock said:

> The method we follow here is to get the patient rapidly under the influence of very large doses. We give three to five grain pills three times a day for three days, one pill after meals for three days; the next three days ten grain pills., the next fifteen; the next 20; and the next 25; so that for three days at the summit of this period, the patient gets 75 grains of Blaud's mixture a day.

With that treatment a man with 50% hemoglobin may reach 80% by the end of two weeks and have normal blood in four weeks. Sometimes, however, posthemorrhagic anemia is incurable, for prolonged anemia paralyzes the blood-forming organs.

Transfusion

On March 31, 1908, Dr. Hoover of Cleveland, "one of the strongest internists in the country,"[9] was in Ann Arbor to address the county medical society, and Dock persuaded him to give a clinic. Hoover discussed a woman with metastases following breast surgery. She had been anemic. Hoover stated: "Dr. Crail [= Crile][10] has been making experiments in transfusion of blood from one patient to another who has sarcoma, and it was noticed directly the transfusion was made there was tremendous jaundice, and very marked haemolysis with haemoglobinaemia and fatal termination within a very short time." Transfusion had been direct from the radial artery of the healthy person to a vein of the recipient. Hoover said that "the blood of the patient had a haemolytic effect on the blood that was introduced, so the addition of the normal blood was a menace to life, in fact cost this patient her life." Hoover described experiments in cross-matching blood of a normal person with blood of a patient with malignancy. He concluded that "there comes a period in malignant growths in which the serum has not only a haemolytic property on the red blood cells of the normal individual, but later there comes a time when the relationship of the red blood corpuscles of the malignant patient is diminished to the normal individual. . . . In what the haemolysis consists is a very obscure thing."[11] There is no evidence that transfusion was attempted at Michigan in Dock's time.

Pernicious Anemias

Dock said his interest in pernicious anemia had been aroused by Pepper, Osler and Musser and that chance had thrown a considerable amount of clinical material his way.[12] In 1899–1908 he presented more than thirty patients with the possible diagnosis of pernicious anemia to Michigan's fourth-year class.

When a student described a lemon-yellow patient with a red cell count of 1,390,000, Dock asked:

What is there in the history that throws light on the condition?

STUDENT: First of all the slow onset and it starts with gastrointestinal symptoms and then he becomes gradually weaker and has syncope and palpitations of the heart on exercise; and then numbness in the extremities.

The student had not made a blood smear, but Dock made the diagnosis of pernicious anemia on the basis of the history. Other doctors may not have made it because they did not examine the blood. Dock stated:

> It is no accident that we see in this clinic so many cases of pernicious anemia. They are scattered all over the country and come into every doctor's office, and the reason they are not more frequently called by that name is that many are called leukemia, many jaundice, many liver disease, and many such harmless terms as general debility, dyspepsia, stomach trouble and so on.

Characterizing the anemia was no problem. Further, "[s]uspecting from the appearance of the skin anemia, it ought not take more than half a minute to bring out all the features that show except the staining and with the right staining, at the outside, not more than five minutes." At that time Dock was using Wright's stain, and the stenographer may have misunderstood what he said.

Red cell counts ranged from as low as 600,000 to 2,670,000, and the color index was high. Leucocyte counts were normal or low, but the cells were abnormal, showing, Dock said, breakdown of the nucleus. Students observed smears under oil immersion. The red cells, "instead of collecting in rolls—all medical students like to say rouleaux—they are bunched up in groups." Students saw poikilocytes and megaloblasts characteristic of pernicious anemia. "But from the character of the reds it would have been a very sporting proposition to say nucleated reds would be found inside of six covers, but we found them in two."

A patient had 14% hemoglobin, and Dock asked: "Has she secondary anemia that has produced pernicious anemia, or has she secondary anemia because she has pernicious anemia?" Such patients usually had complete absence of hydrochloric acid from the stomach. Dock said:

> Some cases of pernicious anemia have been said to be due to atrophy of the stomach or mucous membrane of the stomach or small intestine and the atrophy looked upon as the etiological factor; but in nearly every case the HC1 is greatly diminished or more often absent so that the results of the test meal are interpreted frequently as being due to the anemia rather than as being the primary factor, that is, the stomach condition looked upon as secondary to the blood condition.

Dock always examined a patient's mouth and teeth, and when he discovered pyorrhea alveolaris in a patient with pernicious anemia he said:

From that we might suspect he has an early condition of indigestion or dyspepsia that would have accounted for the disease; but whether this is true or not it is not always easy to make out. Dr. Hunter of England says that in most cases there is an inflammation of the mouth and that he looks upon as the primary condition and thinks the disease starts from stomatitis.[13] If that is the case, it seems rather queer that there aren't more cases of pernicious anemia because 75 per cent. of the cases we get in the hospital here have inflammation of the mouth, especially about the gums, whereas the percentage of cases of pernicious anemia, as you know is small.

Dock also dismissed worry as a cause for a similar reason.

STUDENT: [A patient with 1,280,000 red cells] has been worrying and getting weaker ever since he contracted his case of gonorrhea last December.

DOCK: Do I understand your attribute the pernicious anemia to worry from gonorrhea?

STUDENT: There doesn't seem to be any particular cause for it.

DOCK: That is partly characteristic of pernicious anemia. But we sometimes find dyspepsia was the direct cause and sometimes worry, that is, worry about financial trouble; worry about gonorrhea is not a common cause, otherwise pernicious anemia would be much more common than it is, and at an earlier stage in life.

Dock said that because the disease is given the name "pernicious" is no reason to say that the prognosis is not hopeful. Nevertheless, he had never seen a recovery. A patient's life may be prolonged by rest, open air, cold douches, massage and a good diet of meat, fruit, and milk. Give him plenty of hydrochloric acid to act as a gastric and intestinal antiseptic. Raw eggs chopped together with raw meat, onions, salt, and pepper make a nourishing dish. Do not give the patient whiskey, but if he does not like his food, he may be given weak alcoholic drinks, claret or sherry or port. Even if he is a teetotaler when well, these make him feel better and improve his appetite. Many studies have shown that iron does no good, but Dock believed in giving arsenic or even bichloride of mercury. Arsenic may turn the patient brown and contribute to his peripheral neuritis, and Dock said it did not reach the seat of the disease. Cushny was skeptical.[14] However, Dock prescribed arsenic for pernicious anemia patients all the time he was in Ann Arbor. When a student said he would give nux vomica and Fowler's solution to a patient with pernicious anemia,[15] Dock asked:

What do you think Fowler's solution does to him?

STUDENT: A theory is that this condition is due to hemolysis, and the Fowler's solution acts antagonistic to the toxins of the blood.

But Dock said that arsenic is toxic to the bone marrow and thereby stimulates red cell production.

Even if we can't explain how arsenic does good, there are many reasons why we ought to keep on using it, the chief reason being that the patients get well when they use arsenic under this condition when very often they don't get well under any other condition. Everybody who has treated a good many cases will say there are certain patients who the minute they get under the influence of arsenic improve more strikingly than patients with any other condition, so the clinical reasons for using it are extremely strong; case after case improves that before had not improved.

Some patients had remissions under Dock's care, and he predicted that one who did would not be alive in five years. The usual course was downhill. A patient with a red cell count of 2,000,000 when first seen had a count of 600,000 four months later. Dock said: "There is nothing to do but temporize. I am afraid the prognosis is as bad as it could be. When you get down below 800,000 it is that the prognosis is the same, no matter what the details are."

Worms and Anemia

In April 1904 a pale, sallow outpatient with a distended abdomen was hastily examined. A blood sample contained red blood cells of diverse shapes, and Dock thought the patient might have pernicious anemia or cancer of the stomach. Three days later he showed the class smears of the patient's blood. Megaloblasts twice the size of red blood cells clinched the diagnosis of pernicious anemia. Dock said: "It wouldn't do if he were a Finn and had just come from that oppressed country. If he were from that country we would have to think of a tape worm infection, the bothriocephalus; or we might think he could have ankylostoma infection, though that is not so common, and he would not be so likely to have such a typical anemic blood." In any case, his stool should be examined for worms.

Just before the class graduated in 1908, Dock gave a long discourse on intestinal parasites, and he said:

> We are fortunate in having today a number of preparations of worms useful to look at and to refresh your minds before going out into the darkness of practice. For example, here are the links of the bothriocephalus latus. We find it usually among Scandinavian people or those along the Baltic sea or the Swiss or South Germans from Bavaria. But it is found in this country, and in Texas, for example, it is believed that it occurs native. It is most important on account of its relation with anemia, although not every patient with *Bothriocephalus* has anemia; in fact, more patients haven't anemia than have, when they have this kind of worm.

Misdiagnosis of Leukemia

Dock said: "In leukemia if we examine the patient even very briefly and very simply, we can make a positive diagnosis. This depends on the fact that leukemia usually comes to our notice when the disease is well established." The diagnosis was frequently missed because physicians had not made an adequate physical diagnosis and had not studied the patient's blood. Appearance might be deceptive.

STUDENT: I don't think he looks as though he had leukemia.

DOCK: Do you think you can tell from a patient's look whether he has leukemia? How do they look?

STUDENT: Like a person with anemia, I think.

DOCK: That is a curious fact that they don't. They look just as he does, with a very red face. All the cases sent down here with a diagnosis of leukemia based on looks turned out to have something else, and the leukemics nearly always were taken for something else.

A patient was sent to the University Hospital with a diagnosis of ovarian tumor. When Dock and the students palpated her abdomen they found the mass was the spleen, not an ovary, not an omental sarcoma, not a pancreatic tumor and not the liver, although the liver is sometimes on the left. Dock said that in this part of the country an enlarged spleen is likely to be a sign of leukemia, in the tropics of malaria. Examination of a blood smear confirmed the diagnosis of leukemia. Dock said: "In one-half such cases the doctor tells the patients that they have ovarian cysts and that after a somewhat simple and ordinary operation they can go home cured. So it was in this case."

A patient with leukemia might be deaf. Dock said: "Patients not knowing they had leukemia have gone to ear clinics and have been punctured and if they got a few drops of oedematous fluid they would say the diagnosis [of otitis media] is correct." But it might be the other way around. Once slides were sent to Dock with the request that he confirm the diagnosis of leukemia. He thought infection more likely and telegraphed the referring physician: "How about the ears?" The doctor replied: "I had just opened one ear drum when your telegram came, and found a free discharge of muco-pus." Dock said failure to examine the ears is malpractice.

In an attempt to decrease the incidence of misdiagnosis, Dock gave a long and detailed lecture to the Washtenaw and Jackson County Medical Societies on May 23, 1905, in which he presented a patient with myelogenous leukemia, one with Banti's disease, and one with pernicious anemia. All three had previously been presented to the fourth-year class in the same detail.

Diagnosis of Leukemia

Dock said that formerly the diagnosis of leukemia was made only when the white cell count was up to 80,000. Now it could be made on the basis of the form of the lymphocytes, and he had made the correct diagnosis when the count was only 1,000. There are signs of degeneration in the nuclei: "little lumps that otherwise do not differ very much in size and shape from the nucleus of normal lymphocytes," or the nucleus may be notched. One can find degenerate cells in a person who looks perfectly well and a few months afterward shows serious changes.[16]

Differential counts were routinely made on blood smears, and a typical report by a student was: "It shows a large number of granular myelocytes, mast cells, basophile polynuclears; I could not find any eosinophiles. It shows poikilocytes, nucleated red, normoblasts." By 1900, Dock said, leukemia was recognized as a disease of the bone marrow as well as of the spleen, and in one instance he said they would have to look in the urine for "a peculiar form of albumin, one that dissolves on heating with nitric acid, although it coagulates when the temperature gets down to 55 C."

Lymph Glands

Many patients had masses in the neck, axilla or groin. Students said they were the size of hens' eggs or robins' eggs, filberts, brazil nuts, hickory nuts or little lima beans. Just once one said: "It is 4″ long and 2″ wide." Dock had his students determine whether the masses were encapsulated and discrete or confluent and whether they were freely movable. When he asked a student to describe their consistency, Dock said. "Consistency means consistency, that is, is it hard, soft, elastic, or non-elastic, brawny or doughy or stringy?"

The differential diagnosis was difficult. One patient had many masses on the left side of her neck and in the axilla. Some were ulcerating.

STUDENT: I think she has chronic tuberculous adenitis or Hodgkin's disease.

DOCK: Are those the only possibilities?

STUDENT: It may be lympho-sarcoma.

DOCK: Why did you not mention that first?

STUDENT: The blood findings indicate it is more likely Hodgkin's.

DOCK: Why?

STUDENT: Because it shows anemia and no leukemia.

DOCK: What does the blood show?

STUDENT: Reds, 3,720,000; whites 30,000; hemoglobin 47 per cent.

DOCK: Why doesn't that indicate Hodgkin's?

STUDENT: Anemia is characteristic of that.

DOCK: Well, we have anemia, but couldn't a patient with lympho-sarcoma have anemia; couldn't a patient with tuberculous glands have anemia? How can you tell? For example, if she had 30,000 leucocytes and all were lymphocytes, what then?

STUDENT: It would be Hodgkin's.

DOCK: If 85 per cent. were polynuclear, what then?

STUDENT: It would show a pyogenic process.

Dock said that if the swelling had come on in the last two or three months, the cause was likely to be tuberculosis; if it had lasted for five years, it was something else again.

Now Hodgkin lived at a time when no one examined the blood, at least histologically, and so it is very likely that Hodgkin included cases of tuberculosis, cancer, sarcoma and a number of other things. The conception of Hodgkin's disease is a very unsatisfactory one. There are some people that believe that Hodgkin's disease is a sort of blood disease. Again other people believe that Hodgkin's disease is simply a name given to a good many kinds of enlarged lymphatic glands.

When a student said he had taken it for granted that the enlarged glands were tuberculous, Dock told him:

But, my dear friend, you must never take anything for granted in a clinical way; or a better way would be to say: "I take it for granted this is tuberculosis, but perhaps I am wrong, let me look it up somewhere." If you had studied you would have found a large number of cases of enlarged glands under thirty different names, and that shows how obscure they are.

Such questions could be settled by biopsy. "[In practice] select one of the easiest, make a hypodermic injection of cocaine, then a short incision and see what you have." When that was done:

[B]ut the point is this: can you make a histological examination and say whether it is tuberculosis, ordinary sarcoma, or a lymphosarcoma, and if a lymphosarcoma, can you tell whether it belongs to that particular type of lymphosarcoma that is known as the Dorothy Reed type—I suppose if Miss Reed's name had been anything else it would have been known as the Dr. Reed type.[17]

When a biopsy was done, a student reported the findings: "hyperplasia of the cells, no giant cells, no new cells."

Prognosis and Treatment

Members of his village had taken up a collection to send a sixteen-year-old boy with an enormously distended abdomen to Ann Arbor for operation. The student responsible reported that the boy's blood contained 1,320,000 red cells and 96,000 white cells with a large percentage of myelocytes, eosinophils, "and I think a few megaloblasts." Dock demonstrated that the mass in the abdomen was an enlarged spleen. The boy's nose bleeds, Dock said, prohibited operation, and the prognosis was poor.

The only criticism I would make is that the doctor [at home] did not keep up the patient's and the family's hopes long enough. If you fail to tell people, on the one hand, that the patient is incurable, they will find it out sooner or later and you will lose your reputation for veracity. If you give up too soon, they will lose confidence in you and go to somebody else.

Dock repeatedly advised students to cultivate skill in prognosis.[18] If they did, they would not be surprised by anything that happened, and they would impress their patients with their acumen.

Dock seldom advised splenectomy because most patients died of the operation. "The operation could only lead to discredit on the part of the doctor." A Mayo, "one of the most competent men in the country," had performed radical excision of enlarged glands on a patient subsequently seen by Dock, but Dock did not recommend the operation. "But on the other hand, point out [to the patient] that while the disease is serious and prognosis nearly always bad, a great deal can be done by treatment."

Dock said that H. C. Wood, his teacher of materia medica at Pennsylvania, was iconoclastic, but Wood had written: "Our knowledge of the value of arsenic in disease rests solely upon clinical observation which abundantly established its use in certain very diverse affections."[19] Dock relied upon his own clinical experience, and throughout his time in Ann Arbor he prescribed large doses of arsenic for his leukemic patients. From at least 1900 he also used X-ray therapy, but he wrote in 1904 that "No stronger case can be made for it than for arsenic."[20] Dock told his students:

Then we give x-rays by exploring over the most important seats of the disease two minutes each, and instead of giving those often, which might bring on a very rapid and dangerous breakdown of abnormal tissues, we give them at intervals of a week, carefully watching the blood between. We use a medium hard tube, with the idea of getting the effect in the tissues and not in the skin.

Sometimes an enlarged spleen or gland in the neck did regress for a while.

If we treat them with x-rays there is a good chance of seeing them reduced; they may get smaller almost like magic; but then another important condition about it is that just about the time the patient seems to be quite well, the glands all down and all healed, she suddenly gets severe toxic symptoms and in a few hours ends. . . . Anybody would be likely to feel as if he had assisted at a murder, although the patient might be very willing to have murder carried out on him.

Malaria

Dock had become familiar with the malaria parasite while acting as Osler's laboratory assistant in Philadelphia, and as soon as he arrived in Galveston, Texas, he began to publish on malaria.[21] There was little of the disease, he said, in Galveston itself, but in his first year there he saw thirty patients from the Texas "bottoms." Others came from Mexico and the "notoriously malarial parts of Louisiana." Some arrived on ships from the Caribbean islands. Dock studied in detail the relation of the different forms of the parasites in the blood to each other and to the clinical symptoms as seen in many patients. He thought malaria is transmissible by blood, but he wrote nothing about mosquitoes.[22]

Dock found very little malaria in Michigan, although fevers were frequently diagnosed as malaria by local physicians who did not examine the blood. Dock said a man who had a fever in the winter in Michigan did not have malaria unless he had had a chill and fever the previous summer. In 1902 Dock made an elaborate study of the distribution of mosquitoes in and around Ann Arbor. He wrote: "The summer of 1902, as you are all aware, was remarkable no less for its weather than for the unusual development of mosquitoes. Even in the closely built up parts of the city the insects were so numerous as to make an evening out of doors a most painful experience."[23] Dock collected mosquitoes from puddles in the streets and along the Huron River eight miles to the east and nine miles to the west of the city. Among the many species found, he identified those capable of transmitting malaria, and he was himself bitten by an anopheles mosquito at 6:00 P.M. on the porch of the Washtenaw Country Club. Therefore, Dock said, the relative scarcity of malaria in Michigan was the result not of the absence of the vector, but of the widespread use of quinine. Many physicians treated almost any fever with quinine, and in addition the misdiagnosis of typhoid fever as "typho-malarial fever" was still common in the hinterland.[24]

Dock, of course, did examine the blood, and he taught his students to do so. The only patient with malaria described in detail in the *Clinical Notes* was shown on April 4, 1902, and before the class began Dock showed the malaria organism under the microscope.

> If you look through that microscope you will find just above the center a bluish body with two clear spots, one on the left and the other on the right. Then if you look carefully you will see a dark red spot, perhaps with a tint of purple in it. Notice incidentally that this is a No. 6 lens that you have. If you cannot find the object with a lower power, you cannot say they are not present. Don't get the idea that this is the power we always use.

If you do not have a microscope, give quinine in a therapeutic test no longer than a week. "We hear a great deal about the therapeutic test. It is a very fallacious thing. It has to be used with every possible source of error excluded."

Dock always insisted that a patient's temperature be taken at least as frequently as every two hours, and consequently he was able to describe accurately the cycle of malarial paroxysms and to gauge his treatment accordingly.[25] Give a single dose of quinine to reach maximal effectiveness at once, and give it in the decline of the paroxysm. A dose of 15 grains will cut off the next paroxysm. Examine the blood the next day, and if it contains no parasites, stop quinine until the second week, when 10 grains is to be given to prevent the relapse that will almost certainly occur.

Dock did not like proprietary preparations of quinine, and he recommended that the powder be dissolved in hydrochloric acid, one drop [concentration not specified] to one grain with syrup of ginger to cover the taste. He did not like pills or capsules.

> DOCK: Here is an interesting specimen I would like to call your attention to. What is it? What are they?
>
> STUDENT: Stones.
>
> DOCK: Well, they look like stones; now they come from a patient with gall stones. Do you think they are stones?
>
> STUDENT: The have roughened edges.

DOCK: They look like tablets, don't they? And that is what they are. The tablet method of giving medicine is extremely popular, . . . but every now and then we see evidence of some weak point about the tablet method of administration and this illustrates one of them and also the need of constant supervision. It is not enough to write a prescription and hand it out, but it is necessary to see that it is being properly taken and properly utilized by the body. On account of just such accidents I have a standing rule never to give tablets, but to give the dry medicine in the form of a powder. . . . [S]ometimes you can find 20 or 30 quinine pills in the intestines of a patient who has not taken any for two or three weeks, lying there, evidently not doing any harm but, on the other hand, not doing any good.

ASCITES

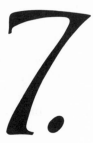

SOMETIMES DOCK AND HIS STUDENTS
could not palpate the spleen, stomach, liver, or kidneys because the abdomen was grossly distended. Then they had to decide whether the abdomen was filled with free fluid, and if it were how the fluid was to be removed. To show how the abdominal contents look in a patient with ascites, Dock once passed around a picture of a cadaver that had been frozen and then sagitally sectioned.[1]

Diagnosis of Free Fluid

On October 9, 1906 Dock began the examination of a patient by saying:

> Now, Mr. Culver, suppose we consider the condition of the abdomen a little. What do you think about it?
>
> STUDENT: I think there is free fluid.
>
> DOCK: I am not at all sure about it; at any rate, we don't begin that way; we first describe what we see and then draw our conclusions afterward. How about the shape? Well, it is greatly distended, isn't it, three or four inches above the level of the thorax; and it is somewhat symmetrical, that is, the two halves have about the same shape and bulge at the sides and that is the thing that may have led you to think of fluid, and it is somewhat flat on the top and that also gives the idea of free fluid in the peritoneum. I don't know how many distended abdomens you may have seen in Dr. Peterson's [obstetric] clinic, but there are so many that have a very different shape so that the abdomen looks almost pear shaped and the sides may not project notably at all; in other cases there is

128

a greater convexity than here but still not the pear shape we see in pelvic tumors of various kinds. But we must not get the idea that in all cases of free fluid we must necessarily have such a shape. But here what we have is a rather characteristic shape for free fluid. The navel is quite full; but neither protrudes nor is it retracted. Where the abdomen is large as the result of fat it is very much retracted. Now what else can we do in order to prove whether there is free fluid?

STUDENT: We can tap him.

DOCK: Well, we can do that, but isn't there some other method we can use?

STUDENT: We can see whether there is fluctuation.

DOCK: Suppose you try that and see. Do you get it? Fluctuation is a thing that when you get a well marked fluctuation it is very easy to recognize. Many that have no free fluid give a wave, either a fat wall or a large soft tumor mass, a large soft fibroid, for example, can produce a very fair fluctuation wave. What else do you think necessary to prove our point?

STUDENT: As the patient sits up the area of dulness would be lower.

DOCK: Suppose you percuss him and see. There you have a tympanitic note. Now how far does it go? Let's see. On the left side it ends at the navel line. The resonance is all down the right side, isn't it? At least it is down in a certain line; that doesn't look as if there was free fluid there. What could produce such a condition? Well, there may be loops of intestine and that is all the more likely finding it on the right side because owing to the way the mesentery is attached, and is there any other possible explanation of it? The fluid may be walled off, but it is all the more important to make careful lines and see where the lines change when we percuss. (Somebody has my good pencil. I would be willing to trade this even for my little one.) (To patient): Suppose you sit up, Mr. *****. (To student): This line here is about right when he lies down. If there is fluid there, of course this line ought to drop, but it really drops very little, doesn't it? But in the middle it becomes dull. (To patient): Now suppose you lie down again. (To student): Suppose we try it from side to side. We note that on this side it is perfectly dull all along the axillary line. (To patient). Now can you roll on your right side? (To student): It is still dull. Let's see how the other line moved. But over here we can't get dulness. Unfortunately, there must be something there that interferes with the free movement of fluid. But the thing to do now is to find out the condition of the fluid in the abdomen and what kind of fluid and, if possible, what is in the abdomen besides fluid. It would be very risky in practice to try to make a diagnosis without knowing what else is there. The ways of finding out are two: the first is to use a needle, stick it through the skin, get the fluid and examine it; another way is to make an incision through the abdominal wall and explore, either with the eye or with the fingers or both of them. In most cases the examination with the knife is to be preferred, for several reasons: first, there is a certain amount of risk about using the needle, when you use a needle you never know where the end is; and, while we use it a thousand times in a year and no error ensues, yet it is an unsurgical way of doing. On the other hand, an incision does not add appreciably to the danger of the operation—there is no greater danger of infecting by incision than by a needle prick, the operation is a trifling one, it can be done under local anaesthesia and if it requires general anaesthesia the risk is rather slight.

When Dock tapped the patient at Monro's point, midway between the umbilicus and the left anterior iliac spine, he obtained 2,450 cc of thin, milky, slightly pinkish fluid of specific gravity 1,014. Its sediment consisted exclusively of lymphocytes. The patient soon died, and at autopsy performed by Warthin a large mesenteric growth continuous with a lymphocytoma of the thoracic duct proved to be the "something that interferes with the free movement of fluid."[2]

Examination of the fluid in similar cases may not reveal how much cancer or tuberculosis exists in the peritoneum, and Dock cited other instances in which the diagnosis had been missed when paracentesis had been done. One was a malignant teratoma that had ascites as its earliest symptom; another was a fibroid tumor of the uterus; and a third was an ovarian fibroid. Dock wrote: "In conclusion, I would not wish to deny the propriety of abdominal paracentesis in all cases. For diagnosis it has a definite field, subject to the limitations I have stated. In treatment, it may at times be useful in inoperable cases, but before beginning this, one should be very sure that a more surgical procedure is out of the question."[3]

Removing Ascitic Fluid

One patient's waist went from 60 inches to 36 inches when she was given a tablespoon of Epsom salts in a glass of water three times a day. Dock said he had hardly ever seen a patient able to take the salts so continuously. Nevertheless, she grew large again, and fourteen quarts of fluid had to be removed from her abdomen.

Dock said the place to tap is "about one-half way between the anterior spine and the navel, but it would not be a proper place to tap if he has intestines there." Gas should be removed from the intestines before tapping, and for this Dock gave saline cathartics. It would be well for students to see the procedure done before attempting it themselves. There is practically no danger, though the patient may faint. If the midline is avoided, a blood vessel probably will not be punctured. Before starting, Dock had the nurse wash the patient's skin, and he asked for a sterile instrument. He said that twenty years before they would simply take one from a drawer, and very few infections resulted.

An interesting point about tapping the abdomen is the remarkable tolerance the peritoneum has about things of this kind. Nobody used to think of having the instrument sterilized, but peritonitis has hardly ever been seen to follow such a thing. There is a case where a man used an ordinary knife, pocket knife, and stuck in the stem of a clay pipe for drainage. I knew of a man who, becoming impatient at the delay of coming of the physician, took a carving knife and stuck it in and drained off several gallons without having any discomfort.

Explore first with a needle; then insert a trocar or make an incision. To incise, freeze the skin with ethyl chloride. "We cut just as the frost goes out and not while the skin is frozen; then the sensibility is still lessened and it is easier to cut."

Dock thought a seventy-year-old man with ascites had cirrhosis of the liver, though he had not used alcohol until a few years ago and then "not more than 5 cents worth of whisky a day." Dock tapped him in class and removed nine liters. While doing so, he said:

> It does no harm to tap the abdomen sitting up, in fact I rather prefer to tap them sitting up because if they get faint, you will discover their faintness more quickly than if you tap them lying down. If there is a tendency to faintness usually the best way to overcome it is by giving the patient a small drink of whisky, not that whisky does any good, but because people are used to looking on whisky as a stimulant.

Sometimes Dock failed: "When you tap high up you may get a string of omentum in your cannula, and the only thing to do is to push it back. There is no harm at all." Then pass a sterile catheter through the cannula. Once when the intestine covered the cannula and Dock got no fluid at all, he said it had happened with this patient before. "I am always—I won't say glad—but take a certain amount of satisfaction in seeing things of this kind fail because that will prepare you for some of the difficulties of practice when you get outside."

Avoiding Trouble at the End of Tapping

Dock showed how to avoid trouble at the end of tapping. The patient was a large Irish woman with cirrhosis of the liver, distended abdomen, edema of the legs and large superficial veins. On a previous occasion Dock had removed a little over twenty liters, but this time tapping was to be done by Dr. McCormick. Dock told the patient: "He comes from the same part of Ireland you do." She said: "If Dr. Dock had not been here I would not have let him touch me." During the exploratory puncture the syringe broke. McCormick inserted a trocar, and while he was at work Dock said: "Have you a bandage? It is better to use a broad bandage. If you tap and run out forty pounds of liquid, there may be a great deal of change in the position of the organs and it is better to compensate that by drawing in the bandage." When McCormick had withdrawn 18,000 cc, Dock thought the old record might be broken. Then:

DOCK.. You haven't had your whisky yet. I think it is time you had some.

PATIENT. God bless Dr. Dock.

DOCK. Happy days.

MOUTH, ESOPHAGUS AND STOMACH

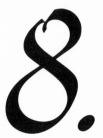

WHEN DOCK PRESENTED THE FIRST
patient of the year on September 28, 1906, he said:

> So here one might begin with the alimentary canal, but that, it is
> always important to remember, begins not at the stomach, but at
> the lips. And when we examine the mouth we see that she has a
> very fine set of teeth in the upper jaw, and they are fine for the rea-
> son that they were bought at a price, but when we examine the
> lower jaw, then what do we see? First, she has very few teeth, five
> all told, or four and a half. One of them is broken off half way
> down, and the most important thing is that those teeth are ex-
> posed for one eighth or one fourth of an inch by retraction of the
> gums. The gums are spongy and around the bottom of the teeth
> there is a sort of greyish exudate looking something like pus, but
> not positively purulent. Such a patient runs the risk of swallowing
> teeth or getting them down the windpipe, and runs the risk of sep-
> tic infection, but aside from that she constantly gets a septic infec-
> tion for every time she swallows she is swallowing some of this
> material.

Her mouth should be washed out with something strong: "Carbolic is
not a nice mouth wash; silver nitrate isn't bad; permanganate is better,
½ per cent.; bichloride, 1 to 10,000 is a good mouth wash. Formalin
would be good if it were not so disagreeable." Brushing the teeth will
make the gums bleed, "but that is just the time when the tooth brush
ought to be used." Dock said:

> Now you may be able to tell me about people you know who have
> very defective teeth and yet are specimens of robust health and I

134

don't deny that such cases exist because I have seen them myself, but that is no more reason for thinking that such a condition is harmless than it is for thinking that because one man can go on smoking 30 or 40 cigars a day or drinking 40 to 50 glasses of whisky a day such a thing is harmless.

Such a patient should be sent to a good dentist. Dentists frequently reciprocate and send their patients to a doctor. Very often a dentist will discover diabetes first. Dock remarked:

> I understand it has been suggested that dentists ought to be doctors. Not wishing to get into the newspapers, nevertheless I would suggest that all doctors had better become dentists; it would do more good to the race if all doctors were dentists than all dentists doctors; unless the doctor has both points of view he may, in fact very often does overlook a very important part of the body.

Obstruction of the Esophagus

In Dock's seventeen years in Ann Arbor he saw thirty-two instances of esophageal obstruction among about five thousand patients on his medical service. Spasm was responsible for obstruction in six of the patients, cancer of the esophagus for sixteen and cancer of the stomach or cardia for seven.[1]

Spasm of nervous origin, Osler had said, usually occurs in women, hysterical patients or those with marked neurotic tendency. "The condition is rarely serious."[2] One of Dock's students agreed with Osler when he described a woman unable to swallow solid food:

> STUDENT: It is a functional disturbance. I think it is mind acting on matter.
>
> DOCK: You must belong to Mrs. Eddy's sect.
>
> STUDENT: I don't belong to any sect, but I believe in the correlation of mind over matter.

The patient, whose inability to swallow had come on suddenly three weeks before, was being fed by rectum "with the idea that the spasm, if spasm is there, may relax with perfect rest."

When obstruction was anatomical, Dock began by auscultating as the patient swallowed water. "In an ordinary individual you hear two murmurs on swallowing; here for a good many seconds nothing could be heard, and then after that a little gurgling sound." Then he explored the patient's throat with his finger. Once he found a thickening back of the middle of the cricoid cartilage; some blood came away from the slightly ulcerated surface. More often he attempted to pass a stomach tube, and he always used a soft one. "Never in the beginning with a hard instrument like an oesophageal bougie." As he passed a tube he described what he felt: "I have passed the cricoid which is always a narrow point, and gives a good many doctors the chance to make a diagnosis of spasmotic stricture and thereby curing it with electricity." When he found an obstruction at the cardia, Dock said: "Now notice that I am beginning to get something although it is about two inches above the cardiac end, unless the patient has an unusually short oesophagus or the tube is too long." He recovered uncoagulated milk that had not been in the stomach, and as he pushed the tube it doubled up. He remarked: "This brings up an extremely important point. It shows the advantage in general of using a large instrument on hollow cavities. If you use a small stomach tube you might easily miss finding what we certainly found, that there is an obstruction at the cardia." When Dock had doubts whether such an obstruction was functional or organic, he said: "I certainly think he ought to be examined with an oesophascope before going further. We will see to that in the morning." The examination would be made by Roy Bishop Canfield, the professor of otolaryngology, who was expert with the instrument.

For treatment Dock passed an olive-pointed whalebone sound, beginning with a small one and then larger and larger ones. He cautioned his students that it "is always well to inspect the first time you use it in a season because they have a way of getting split or cracked." The work requires patience. Dock said, "or there are sounds that are made to be separated that can be put down through the obstruction and then opened up, or you can put a permanent sound in and the solid sound will gradually soften up the tissue so that the orifice will become larger."

More often Dock referred such patients to a surgeon who might make a gastrostomy and dilate the obstruction from below or excise it if possible. A surgeon should have permission to do any possible operation. There was always the question of advisability of operation:

DOCK: He says "What would you do?"

STUDENT: If it would prolong my life, I would have it done.

DOCK: That is the proper way to answer. It seems to me, however, although I am rather given to advising other people to be operated, if I had a thing of that kind and could get a certain amount of food down, with the aid of a stomach tube or otherwise, I would let the thing go.

Stomach Trouble

A patient had vomited first "white stuff" and then "green stuff." Dock said the first was mucus and saliva and the second was bile. "It indicates merely severe vomiting. Always remember that although we might say that there is antiperistalsis there, yet that is rather fanciful. Bile is present in the duodenum only a few inches below the stomach and violent vomiting can easily force the bile into the stomach mechanically." Dock passed around a sample of the vomitus so that students could recognize the fishy smell of bile. He also said that the stomach is frequently ruptured by vomiting, and then there is blood in the vomitus.

Another patient had had a very large gastric hemorrhage three weeks before.

DOCK: Where does the hemorrhage come from?

STUDENT: From the stomach.

DOCK. Did you look that up in the book?

STUDENT. No, I thought it was the stomach.

DOCK: The book saves you the trouble of thinking. What does the textbook say about the relation between the splenic vessels and a hemorrhage from the stomach? You will find that there is a close relation between the stomach veins and the splenic veins. The stomach veins become enlarged and form little varices on the stomach wall, and sometimes they rupture and a hemorrhage follows. This I say is one of the most important causes for a large gastric hemorrhage, especially when we find an enlarged spleen and anemia.[3]

It was not safe to pass a stomach tube. The patient was operated upon for a fibroid tumor by Dr. Peterson. She died a month after the operation as the result of hemorrhage from an eroded gastric varix.

Sometimes gastric disease could be discovered by inspection.

STUDENT: I don't see anything particular about his face.

DOCK. You don't?

STUDENT: He is flushed over the cheeks and nose.

DOCK: Is it flush or something else?

STUDENT: The capillaries are dilated.

DOCK: You might say the venules are dilated. Whenever you see such a thing, although you realize the patient may have been a hard drinker, yet such a thing is always suggestive of stomach disease. That is, the patient has a stomach facies. When you see such a thing, never stop until you examine the patient's stomach. . . . Anybody who would try to treat a person without becoming perfectly familiar with the stomach workings would be as guilty of negligence as a person who in an obstetrical case failed to make out the condition of the urine. In that case anybody can see whether the doctor has been negligent or not. In the stomach cases nobody knows but the doctor and his colleagues, so if he neglects such cases, he has only his own conscience, provided he has the remnants of such a thing left, to indicate that he has been doing wrong.

Chemical Tests of Gastric Function

In 1904 Dock showed the students the form, devised by his colleague David Murray Cowie, for recording the results of gastric analyses.[4] "It

DEPARTMENT OF INTERNAL MEDICINE

STOMACH EXAMINATION

Date ...Name in full...Test meal employed...Time in stomach...
General Character.—Quantity.......c. c....Lavage after..........
    odor ....color................bile.............
    blood, macroscopic ....occult...................
    remains from previous meal ....
    mucus ....
Microscopic Characters.—Blood corpuscles......Leukocytes........
    fragments of mucosa...................Specimen No........
    sarcinæ ....yeasts........moulds........protozoa........
    epithelial cells ....
    fragments of mucosa...................Specimen No.......
Filtrate ....quantity.......color.......specific gravity........
    Reaction.—Litmus ....Congo red....................
    Hydrochloric acid.—Günzberg ....
        dimethyl-amido-azo-benzole ....
    Lactic acid.—Uffelmann ....Kelling.............
        ether extract ....Method.............
    Acetone.—In distillate, Lieben...........Gunning............

(a) Free HCl	....	=	....% gms....Method
(b) Loosely combined HCl.	....	=	....% gms....Method
(c) Organic acids and acid salts	....	=	....% gms....Method
(d) Total acidity..........	—	=	

    Lactic acid % ....
Digestion Tests.—Pepsin, millimeter digested sq. =................
    P. V. Computed for 10 hrs =.........................
    Pepsinogen, millimeter digested sq =........................
    P. V. Computed for 10 hrs =.........................
    Chymosin ....
    Chymosinogen ....
Proteid digestion.—Primary albumoses.........................
    Secondary albumoses ....Peptons.............
Starch digestion ....
    Starch (dark blue)........amylodextrin (lighter blue)........
    erythrodextrin, violet blue....violet....red violet....red......
        mahogany brown ....
    achroodextrin, anachrom ....
    Maltose ....Dextrose ....
Absorption Test—KI reaction occurred in........................
Motor Power Test.—Salol reaction occurred in...................
    Remarks ....
        Examined by.............................

FIGURE 11. Form used in Dock's department for reporting gastric analyses.

works out very well for diagnostic and therapeutic purposes." Dock gave a lecture occupying nine pages of transcript on how to make the analyses, but he ended by saying that he did not "expect anybody to remember all these solutions. . . . I would rather condition a man for remembering it. You need a book and a book like Dr. Novy's laboratory book ought to answer the purpose." Novy, who was responsible for teaching physiological chemistry as well as bacteriology, had already drilled the students in quantitative chemical methods for analysis of saliva, gastric juice, pancreatic juice, and bile.[5] In addition, Arneill's book contained a full description of Dock's clinical laboratory methods for studying the stomach.

The Technique of Gastric Analysis

Dock said many tests were made without adequate preparation, and food is recovered when the stomach tube is first passed.

> DOCK (reading notes): "40 c.c. were recovered and food remains were found." It is always instructive to consider the character of notes and to see how important it is to have notes clear; for example, "food remains." No doubt the man who made the note knows what he means but he should state what kind, that is vegetable tissue, meat or what else.

Consequently, the stomach must be washed out before the test is done. Dock demonstrated the funnel through which water is poured into the stomach tube. Once while he was pouring water:

> DOCK: Do you think you could lie flat on your back?
> PATIENT: You want to kill me.

The wash fluid was emptied by the patient bearing down or by aspirating with a bulb.

Dock said the stomach is not sterile. The motility, not the hydrochloric acid, keeps bacteria low. If motility is reduced, as it is in cancer of the stomach, lactic acid accumulates. Dock asked: "Well, do you ever get lactic acid in a healthy stomach? If you had studied physiology in the dark ages of about twenty years ago you would have learned that lactic acid was one of the normal digestive acids. It is not a normal acid, but it depends upon two things: first, bacterial growth; second, changes in the food."

Culture methods, Dock said, are not worth the trouble clinically. Lactic-acid-producing Oppler-Boas bacilli can be identified in smears. Some said the presence of Oppler-Boas bacilli is positive evidence of cancer of the stomach, but both Dock and Arneill thought they were frequently found in nonmalignant conditions. Lactic acid in gastric concents is identified by Kelling's test: diluted gastric juice is treated with one or two drops of an aqueous solution of ferric chloride. A distinct greenish yellow color is seen when the solution is held up to the light. Consequently, it is important to wash the stomach out thoroughly before making a test for lactic acid production, and the Boas meal containing no lactic acid is given. To prepare that meal, add a teaspoon of rolled oats to one liter of water, and boil the mixture down to 500 cc.

In those days the Ewald meal was standard elsewhere: 35 to 75 grams of white bread with the crust removed, chewed thoroughly and washed down with 350 cc of weak tea. Dock preferred Michigan breakfast foods: granose or shredded wheat.

> The patient can be given a shredded wheat biscuit, which is a very convenient test breakfast for a number of reasons. In the first place, it has nothing in it but wheat, the condition is very uniform, so it isn't like bread which varies in consistency in different places. Then the shredded wheat usually does not have to be weighed, and it is also a thing that can not be swallowed without a certain amount of chewing. He can wash the bread down with water, but it is difficult to wash down shredded wheat biscuits; so the patient nearly always follows your advice, which you should always give: —to chew it thoroughly and sip the water from time to time.

Motor power of the stomach is judged by the volume of gastric contents recovered at the end of an hour.

For measurement of hydrochloric acid, 10 cc of a filtrate of recovered gastric contents is titrated with decinormal sodium hydroxide solution. Titration to the end point of Töpfer's reagent [pH 3.5] gives "free acid," and titration to the phenolphthalein end point [pH approximately 8] gives "total acid." "Combined acid" is the difference between the two.

The results were invariably reported as numbers without units. Once a student said he did not understand why the titration was multiplied by 10. Dock explained that one titrates 10 cc, but wants to know how much decinormal NaOH is required for 100 cc. As Dock said: "There is a practical advantage to that. The results are not absolutely correct. . . . We are working with certain quantities that have a fairly even ratio looked at in large figures and that is the reason it is better [to multiply the volume of NaOH used]. It looks exact and strictly scientific to put it in decimal function, but it isn't." Nowhere did Dock give evidence of recognizing that the number obtained is the millinormality of the solution.

Passing the Tube

In 1905 Dock wrote: "Out of the many thousands examined, I have encountered only two people in whom I could not successfully use the stomach tube at first trial."[6] The quotation demonstrates either Dock's extreme assiduity or his carelessness with numbers. If passing a stomach tube and recovering gastric contents occupied a minimum of fifteen minutes, Dock had spent 31.25 eight-hour days at that task alone for each thousand tests he had performed.

Dock did have trouble:

There are two kinds of patients: those who know all about it from seeing friends or relatives use [the stomach tube]; other people who have heard about it and declare they will never take [it], sometimes a whole population will declare that it is a fearful instrument. In this particular patient six weeks ago I got the tube down three times and telling him to breathe, he absolutely wouldn't breathe. Usually when you tell a patient to breathe he automatically breathes, but this patient had such a fixed idea about the tube he did not pay any attention to my command, and absolutely did not breathe from the time the tube touched his mouth until he pulled it out with great force.

Dock told of another patient who chewed holes in the tube "and the acrobatic tricks that he did while I was passing it would have been great in any show."

A patient might vomit: "Now in passing the tube it is much more comfortable to have a Mackintosh, but on the other hand, you do not need a Mackintosh; with two towels one over the back and the other over the front parts of the body." There might be trouble with the tube: "This tube is coiled; one should keep a stomach tube in such a way that they will be straight. Why is this kept coiled? That is a thing that never should be allowed to happen." Once a student thought the blood found in gastric contents was the result of accidental wounding by the tube. Dock remarked: "That often happens by rough handling of the tube. A tube with a sharp edge around the hole should not be used for ordinary purposes; it is better to have the windows in the tube smooth. Round them off with a hot wire. You should not pass the tube the first time you see a patient, not so much because of the danger but because if anything did happen, accusations of abruptness would be hard to disprove."

Results of Gastric Analysis: Hyperchlorhydria

Dock did not rely on a single test meal. Often results of three meals were reported, and once there were six. When total acidity in three successive meals was 90, 82, and 70, a student said the decrease was the result of treatment. Dock said that was simply normal variation, hence the need for more than one test. Hyperchlorhydria could not be diagnosed unless free acid is greater than 70.

When Dock attempted to find the cause of hyperchlorhydria in a patient whose total acid was 105, he said:

It is not a primary disease, but nearly always comes from something else,—whether there is something wrong with the gray part of the cortex or the appendix or gall bladder,—we cannot always tell, but that as a primary or so-called idiopathic disease, hyperchlorhydria does not account for very much. We look around, first for one of the common sources of hyperchlorhydria, namely some anomaly of the eye, whether muscle weakness or refractive error.

Hyperacidity is associated with headaches, severe neurasthenia and, in the male, functional impotence. Dock sometimes diagnosed "hyperacidity from nervous trouble rather than organic disease." A patient may be in "a general neurotic state," or neurosis affecting the stomach may be a reflex from dropped organs: enteroptosis or nephroptosis. In the female it is sometimes the result of displacement of the pelvic organs.

A student attempting to distinguish among gastritis, gastric ulcer, a neoplasm or gastric neurosis favored neurosis.

DOCK: Why?

STUDENT: All the organs, such as the kidneys and spleen are readily palpable, and the stomach is enlarged and is felt considerably below the umbilicus, the right kidney is slightly movable, and the patient gives a histroy of nervousness before marriage and there is a history in the family of similar conditions that might account for it.

DOCK: Then to go a little further you are quite right in saying that these various displacements have a good deal to do with the neurotic condition. First they act by affecting the patient reflexly. Or the patient may be affected directly or indirectly by knowing she has such an unnormality. We never ought to tell a person with a floating kidney or prolapse of the stomach unless it is absolutely necessary. Formerly we always used to recommend such a person have them sewed up and usually they were just as bad afterward as before and sometimes a great deal worse.

Dock was echoing Osler who had written that sometimes the symptoms of enteroptosis or nephroptosis date from knowledge of that condition.[7] In this instance Dock recommended fattening the patient so that perirenal fat would hold the kidney in place.

Hyperchlorhydria could be controlled by washing out the stomach with tepid water containing Carlsbad salts and then with cool water to remove the alkaline salt. When Dock washed out a patient's stomach, he said: "You want to get the patient to move about while you are washing. If on a table, have him move first on one side and then on the other, have him stand up, so that the water is in contact with all parts of the stomach." Some patients became addicted to gastric lavage. One woman washed her stomach out every night between nine and ten o'clock with four or five quarts of water, and Dock had her demonstrate how much water her stomach would hold.

If a patient objects to repeated gastric lavage, bismuth can be prescribed. Some patients say they have taken barrels of carbonate of soda, and Dock advised students to use that if they were called to a house in the country. Murray Cowie had read Pavlov's recently translated book,[8] and he knew that the secretory response to a protein meal is greater than to a carbohydrate meal. Consequently, Dock suggested a patient cut down on the amount of meat in his diet. Cowie had also learned that fat inhibits gastric secretion in experimental animals. In an elaborate series of experiments on thirty-two University Hospital patients, he had found that one or two ounces of olive oil given just before or with a meal reduces acid secretion and delays emptying.[9] He also found that olive oil given after the meal does not affect previously occurring secretion. Therefore, Dock recommended olive oil before meals "in the way so carefully worked out by Dr. Cowie. . . . Cottonseed oil is just as good and what most of us use when we think we are using olive oil. In Germany they use linseed oil."

Gastric Ulcer

X rays and a contrast medium were never used for diagnosis of gastric ulcer in Dock's time in Ann Arbor. He made the diagnosis on the basis of the history: intense pain in the stomach region that is relieved by food and then comes on again at the height of digestion. "If people have a sharply localized pain in the epigastrium they usually point to it with one finger. If the patient has a diffuse pain he is likely to put the whole hand over it." There may be occult blood in the stool, but often the stool looks like tar.

In 1908 a student described the symptoms a patient had had for twenty years: tarry stools after vomiting blood. The patient was gray, for he had been taking silver nitrate as a styptic.

DOCK: When you say gastric how do you know it is gastric rather than duodenal? What are the symptoms?

STUDENT: Pain coming on three or four hours after meals, relieved by eating. He is also bothered with it nights too.

DOCK: Isn't that rather suggestive of ulcer of the duodenum? What have you to say about the relative importance of differential diagnosis of ulcer of the stomach and duodenum?

STUDENT: I think it does not matter much.

DOCK: Why not?

STUDENT: The treatment is about the same.

Dock dropped the subject without further comment.

One patient with severe vomiting said he had thrown up a gallon of bloody fluid. Dock said.

In the first place we never believe that all the bloody stuff people talk about has been blood. Experience shows that this is almost invariably true, no matter where the blood comes from. We are always told the quantity is larger than it really is. If a man loses a gallon of blood he loses 1/3 of the blood that he has in his body and he loses it quickly, and he would not only faint at the time but he would be extremely weak and would have a collapsed appearance for two or three days afterward.

Then:

An examination of the stomach is the next thing in order, and the examination with the tube ought to be done with forethought. If she has an ulcer, especially bleeding ulcer, or carcinomatous bleeding, it might be dangerous or inconvenient to examine with a tube. First it might occur that perforation would follow. That would be a very unfortunate accident to happen; it might not have been the tube, but it would be hard to get people not to believe it had been the tube. Still we use the tube over and over again with ulcer or suspected ulcer, and very few doctors have any trouble with it.

Once, when the diagnosis had been in doubt a week earlier, the student said:

The diagnosis is easy now.

DOCK: Now you might think there was some interposition of Providence on our part that made the patient have a hemorrhage.

Had passing the tube brought on the hemorrhage?

DOCK: This accident is likely to happen with everyone using a stomach tube, so one should always be on the watch. What would you do in such a case?

STUDENT: Lay the patient flat on his back first, and if his pulse got weak leave him there and give him aconite. If the heart beat disappeared I would bandage his legs and apply hot water bags to his stomach.

DOCK: Suppose that the patient did not faint. What would you do if just a small amount came up? Yes, that would be the thing to do—go ahead and wash him out with cold water, or, if you have it there, hot water, about 105°. So in a case of that kind you would keep on washing and trying to make out that you were accustomed to that sort of thing.

There might be another cause of hemorrhage.

DOCK: Another thing is his burn. He had a severe burn on his head and after that what did he have? What are patients with burns likely to get?

STUDENT: Gastric or duodenal hemorrhage.

DOCK: Now a few days after his burn he did have a gastric hemorrhage although we can't say positively that it comes from his burn.

Ulcer Treatment

A patient with characteristic ulcer pain and occult blood in his stool had been treating himself for twenty years. Dock remarked: "So we have a patient here who had an ulcer for many years, and for years he was in the habit of rolling himself over a barrel. They have to have, of course, a barrel handy. It seems difficult to understand how they can be relieved, but there is no doubt at all about the fact." Dock discussed other treatment with the students. Should the patient be put to bed, and, if so, for how long? Should his stomach be washed out regularly? Dock did not think that did much good. What kind of diet? Nutritious foods easily digested: raw or soft-boiled eggs, milk with lime water, custard or junket. How is junket prepared? "The directions are on the package so I never try to remember them because it is like a minister trying to remember the Lord's prayer at ceremonies, he nearly always forgets the important part of it." Dock ended by prescribing alkalies, bismuth, silver nitrate and an operation if the patient did not improve.

At another time Dock said:

The most important treatment is the dietetic treatment, that is, the treatment of throwing out the use of the stomach and keeping the patient nourished by nutritive enemata. . . . You will find a great many men scoffing at the idea of rectal feeding and wondering whether it is of any value. The physiological chemist proves in the test tube that there is no food excreted into the bowel. Still you have to feed the patient some way, and milk or some of the peptones don't need to be converted by substances in the bowel, but as such are nourishment. The first thing we have to do to give this is to clean out the bowel thoroughly one hour before we wish to give the nourishment. Then the nourishment is given with the patient lying on one side and with the buttocks on one or two pillows. You might use, say this: Liebig, 150 grams of chopped raw beef; 50 grams chopped pancreas, a little salt; 150 c.c. sterile warm water, and in order to keep it in use, say 15 drops tincture opia. Or the Boas: 250 grams milk, 2 eggs, a teaspoonful of starch, a teaspoonful of salt, wine and considerable albumin. You should never use more than 8 ounces, beginning with four ounces, and there should never be more than four feedings a day, and you should have nurse that knows how to give the feedings; and you should stop for a day at the first sign of things going wrong. Combined rectal with subcutaneous feeding is hard to do in private practice. You can't get your sterile stuff. So if things go badly up above we may have to resort to rectal feeding and everybody should have a few formulae at his tongue's end and know how to use rectal alimentation.

Dock told of a doctor's wife who refused to be fed by rectum.

Surgical Treatment

DOCK: But the more we learn the more we realize that these methods are not always to be depended on, so some advanced stomach experts say that there is no use treating a stomach medically unless you can keep the patient in bed two months. For myself I would not do anything of that kind; the idea of staying in bed two months and then finding the ulcer bleeding just as bad as before would not be according to my choice. If the patient has had ulcer for many months, whether mild or severe, the question comes up whether it would not be necessary to do something more than medical treatment, because the ulcer becomes callous, with hard fibrous walls, 1/4 or 1/2 inch thick, just as thick as gristle, with poor blood vessels and very few, so that healing hardly goes on at all. So that something else becomes necessary, and the method of treatment is by surgical operation. That is, operation will do two things,—put the ulcer at rest, and, in the next place, keep the stomach drained. Most ulcers are near the pylorus or the pyloric end, and thus in a part of the stomach that acts like a sort of a churn or mill, grinding over the food in such a way as can never allow the stomach to get well as long as it is functionating normally. So we have to give what the surgeons call drainage; that is, to make an opening so that the food will go out before it reaches the pylorus and so that it cannot retain the contents. So that the operation is not the removal of the ulcer, but rather the formation of a new outlet which is put in the lower part of the stomach, the posterior wall is the place of choice, and another into the jejunum as high up as possible. When that is done certain things follow: the ulcer heals, the patient has no more vomiting of blood and none in the stools. On the other hand it sometimes happens that vicious circles set up in the dead tissue and symptoms set up from this; or he gets a peptic ulcer in the jejunum. At any rate, he is likely to have his symptoms back again. When the first results of these operations were observed there was a rush as for circumcision when people first discovered about the results of infection, etc., thus; but when people got a larger knowledge it became clear the operation was not so simple and complete as one might hope. So we ask the patient whether he can stand the time and expense of medical treatment with the prospect of not being very well then or whether he prefers to have an operation with a chance of getting absolutely well. Results in this hospital have borne out this fact. We have operated on patients who have had gastric ulcer for from a few months to many years, and some were semi-invalids not able to earn their living. Many have been restored to complete health. Those were the favorable cases.

Distending the Stomach

Dock often distended the stomach for diagnostic purposes, and he said a "very important part of abdominal palpation is to get used to palpating a distended abdomen." One method was to pour in a quart of water and then to find the percussion boundaries, but gas was more frequently used. When there was a question whether a mass in the abdomen was in the stomach, a student said:

I would blow up the stomach with air and see the outline.

DOCK: Distend is a little better word. If you talk of blowing up a man you frighten him.

To inflate his stomach, a patient drank a solution of tartaric acid and then one of sodium bicarbonate. By 1900 Dock preferred inflating through a tube, and air could be removed through the tube at the end. He said that after passing the tube, you can blow up the stomach with your own mouth. That is not very pleasant, and the patient may vomit in your face. "Another device is to have a hole in the tube and have the patient inflate his own stomach. That is ingenious, but I don't think it is very good." In 1905 Dock used a bicycle pump.

An enlarged stomach or a dropped stomach was a common finding. Dock said that in addition, "[q]uite a number of cases of enteroptosis and neurasthenia if severe always show floating 10th rib. If we distend the colon by means of gas the colon is also enlarged; it is M shape. The intestines have really lost their bearings, and the mesentery become very long."

A student suggested that the dropped stomach was caused by the patient's corsets.

STUDENT: Well, you know the corset liver.

DOCK: Yes, I know it very well. The corset liver is a very well recognized condition and in some parts of the world very common; for example in Germany very often you will see an example of corset liver in a p.m. room, but in this country it is rather rare specimen; in especially marked cases in Germany it is cut in two. In this hospital in the last fifteen years we have had three cases of corset liver that could be recognized clinically. I think the difference can be explained form the different style of corset; in this country while they wear them tight, they are not tight in the same way you see them in Germany where they have extremely narrow constriction, and you get not only tightness but a short extent of tightness. As for the supposition that corsets can produce such a complication in the stomach it is extremely far fetched; there are so many dropped stomachs in men and although there are men who are said to wear corsets, I doubt very much if any of our patients here ever wear corsets.

The patient said she wore her corsets only on Sunday. Dock questioned her about how tightly she laced them. Did she fasten the string to the bureau and walk away?

A dilated stomach could be treated surgically by putting folds in it, or more simply with a bandage. Dock suggested: "The ordinary abdominal belt that is prescribed in the gynecological clinic, if the belt is put on while standing up does no good. Put the patient in the knee-chest position before you put on the belt. Then put the belt on and have it good and tight, and frequently the symptoms are relieved."

Detecting Gastric Tumors

In 1900 Dock said that "we must never allow ourselves to exclude malignant disease because the patient has had a benign disease for a long time." A gastric ulcer might turn into cancer; many believed that, but no one had been able to prove it. Five years later when a student suggested that an ulcer was becoming malignant, Dock asked: "Just what proportion show that? Some say 60 per cent., and others none at all and still others give every figure between those extremes. It is probably safe to say, however, that the change doesn't occur in more than two or three per cent., so while we ought to think of it it is not as common as we sometimes imagine."

When an autopsy showed primary carcinoma of the stomach with widespread metastases, Dock asked why the diagnosis had been missed. He had not been able to feel the tumor, but he had failed to recognize the value of the test meal results. Typically there would be long-standing dyspepsia and retention, and 2,000 cc had been recovered from the stomach of one patient when he entered the hospital. Dock said: "Ulceration is one of the natural conditions of a new growth, and you are likely to get what from that? One is blood and the other is pus. You look for evidence of unusual bacterial growth in the stomach. They are likely to grow in a stomach made rough and uneven by a new growth." Dock described some gastric washings the students examined under the microscope: "The most interesting thing about the bacteria of the contents is that the patient has so many germs that wherever you get a drop of the stuff you find it strewn with bacilli so that they present the appearance of a lawn in which the grass has just been cut." Bacteria produce lactic acid, but hydrochloric acid is usually absent.

Dock found a tumor in the epigastric region of an emaciated patient, and he marked its boundaries. Asking a student to palpate, Dock said: "Now just because I made those marks I don't insist on any one else getting the same ones now. There are two possibilities: I might have been wrong in my outline, or the mass may have changed." He continued:

The first thing to do is to get your hands warm. You cannot palpate the abdomen with cold hands. It is out of the question. Then you palpate in parts of the body where you do not expect to find anything. That gives you two advantages. It gives you the idea of the healthier side of the two and you get the abdomen accustomed to palpation so that it does not resist so much. . . . It is always useful to engage a patient in conversation when you are palpating the abdomen because it makes the reflex from the attention less marked and it keeps the mouth open more or less so that you don't get so much strain on the diaphragm. . . . Still another thing that might be done with the patient is to examine him in a hot bath. Immerse the patient in a bath about 100 degrees, and run it up to 110 degrees and in that way relax the abdominal wall, and we would be able to find things that we would not otherwise.

A student who found a small mass said:

There isn't enough of a mass to palpate.

DOCK: You must not wait until the mass gets to be as big as a house. If you feel a local hardness, no larger than a pea, it may be much more important to find it than if it were the size of a cocoanut.

Often the mass was large. Dock said: "It sometimes happens, but not very often, that a patient will have a large mass in the body they know nothing of. If patients have small tumors that they know nothing of, it is not to be wondered at, but it seems strange one can have a mass so large as that without knowing anything about it." Then, is the mass in the stomach? "You might say it was in the stomach for these reasons, it is very superficial, it occupies the position of stomach tumors; a stomach tumor is a common thing, especially in the male; it has the mobility on respiration that stomach tumors often have; it is not oval like the spleen, and does not correspond to the movements of a liver or gall bladder tumor."

On May 6, 1904, Dock said:

We have been trying to do something to a patient here which, if it had worked, would have been interesting for all of us to see, but it has not worked. What we wanted to do was to illuminate his stomach in such a way that we could see whether those masses are in front of the stomach or somewhere else. The way you work is to insert an electric light into the stomach, having the stomach partly filled with fluid. You have the stomach partly filled with water to keep it cool and chiefly for the purpose of giving it shape. Instead of using water, we are using a solution of fluorescein.

The battery was run down, or the contacts were broken.

Dock told the students never to use the word *cancer* in front of a patient.

DOCK: We never ought to speak of a tumor before a patient. Patients have a different idea of tumors than doctors. Patients have an idea if they hear the word tumor that it means malignant disease and particularly carcinoma. Now we can't stop and tell every patient that when we call a thing a tumor it does not necessarily mean a malignant tumor, so it is better to avoid the word altogether, avoid it in the clinic and say "swelling." It doesn't sound so scientific as a tumor but it saves time. (To patient): Have you been at all alarmed by hearing us talk about tumors?

PATIENT: No sir.

DOCK: What did you think we meant or didn't you care?

PATIENT: I didn't care.

DOCK: She is the first patient I have seen for a good many years that would give an answer like that.

Nevertheless, Dock frequently violated his own rule. An example:

DOCK: He has a tumor there that has all the characteristics of cancer of the stomach. No medicine will take that away, nor any method of treatment we know will cure it. The only thing that will probably get rid of it is a surgical operation—but it can't get the secondaries out.

PATIENT: Can I ask a question? You say it will last five or six years. What happens then?

DOCK: Why, what do you mean?

PATIENT: Don't they live longer than that?

DOCK: They get cancer somewhere else. Now, of course, to a man like most of you a matter of five or six years might not seem very great; but with the prospect of only six months ahead of him, five or six years is a great deal of a boon. It is not whether we can give the patient an indefinite life, but whether we can give him anything at all.

Question of Surgery

In 1905 Dock wrote: "With greater care in diagnosis, more accuracy in selection, more skill in applying methods to the conditions, the future will show such advances that gastric surgery will be the first, not the last, refuge in suspected malignant disease."[10]

There was the risk of dying on the table: "Most patients who die under anesthesia are those who have had their hearts examined and nothing found the matter with them. They are accidents that can't be helped or guarded against by care in giving the anesthesia. If you do everything you can to prevent the accident, then you need not worry yourselves about the consequences."

Of an eighty-year-old patient:

STUDENT: I think his age is so advanced that it would not be worth while operating.

DOCK: I think we could leave that to the patient. His age is advanced compared to yours, but I remember a discussion of cancer of the stomach before a medical society. A doctor of seventy years old asked me what I meant by saying that the patient was too old, that if he had cancer of the stomach he wanted to be considered as any other case.

Dock advised early operation:

I hope the patient will be operated. It is unfortunate to see such a patient waiting until it is too late. Such a patient we had about a year ago. He refused an early exploration and when it was too late came back and all we could do for him was to give him a gastroenterostomy, send him home and let him be fed through the opening, and his gratitude at having that done was so great as to teach an important lesson about the value of such cases.

A patient returned three years after Cyrenus Darling had done a palliative gastroenterostomy with enterostomy. She had gained forty pounds. Dock said: "You can get statistics showing recoveries and duration of improvement, but those after all are merely statistics that have very little meaning, but it strikes me that it is very much better if we can find out from a person who has gone through such an experience what she thinks about it." The patient was glad she had had the operation.

THE LOWER
DIGESTIVE TRACT

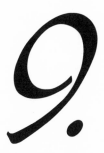

DOCK AND HIS STUDENTS OFTEN HAD
difficulty determining the locus of a mass in the abdomen. Once when
he had failed to diagnose "primary carcinoma of the caecum" that was
revealed at autopsy, Dock asked: "Now the question comes up, how did
we make this mistake? That the exact nature of the patient's growth
wasn't recognized? Was it because it was impossible from the nature of
the mass, or was our observation inexact, or did we draw the wrong
conclusions? All of these come into play." Had the mass been found earlier, it might have been removed, and Dock added that "owing to the
ease of operation nowadays, many people are disinclined to make a
refined diagnosis."

When prolonged palpation failed to define the position of an abdominal mass, Dock distended the colon. It is

> something everybody should learn to do. In order to do that you
> pass the rectal tube connected with a blower of some kind. You in-
> sert the tube as far as you can go, getting it in gently; you ought to
> get it in six or seven inches at the least. If you can get it in a foot, so
> much the better. Push it gently. feeling all the time to see how it
> goes. If it catches, give a little twist, and keep on that way wiggling
> it gently from one side to the other so that the point will not catch
> in the mucous membrane. It is difficult to get the tube through the
> sigmoid flexure, but sometimes you can get it through the splenic
> flexure and over to the hepatic side.

In this instance the student also inflated the stomach. The mass was
found not to be the spleen, and it was in front of the stomach. Dock
drew diagrams on the blackboard to show its relation to the colon.

Ascitic fluid interfering with palpation could be removed by tapping. If distention of the intestine made palpation difficult, a quart of water containing a teaspoon of turpentine mixed with glycerine and soap infused through a rectal tube passed high up might empty the entire alimentary canal. "But it is not well to give too much turpentine. The enema may remain in and the patient absorbing the turpentine, may turn up in a few days with an acute nephritis." Dock did not believe anyone should attempt to remove gas from the intestine by passing a trocar through the abdominal wall.

X rays and a contrast medium were occasionally used. In 1907 Dock said of a man with an enormously distended abdomen: "The man has very interesting x-ray plates that we will see at some time. We tried to get plates after giving him bismuth. The course of bismuth through the intestinal tract is pretty well known now, and we not only see where the bismuth is, but the coils of the intestine. In a good skiagraph we can see them almost as well as if we had the coils before us." Of an earlier patient Dock said everything was pushed together in the abdomen so that ordinary X rays would not go through it. "As it costs $2.50 or $3.00 to try and our account is getting low, I haven't thought it worth while doing that."

The Rectal Examination

Dock did rectal examinations in the afternoon clinic. He thought anemia and paralysis of the blood-forming organs result from bleeding hemorrhoids, but students must learn to look for other problems in the rectum and prostate gland. "One can find cases where patients are being treated for trifling diseases, when they have other and malignant troubles. It is not safe to treat them without examining the rectum." Further, Dock said:

Palpating the rectum is an art that requires a certain amount of practice. In the beginning there is always the trouble about the contraction of the sphincter on the finger. Some of them contract so tightly that you have hardly any sensation left in it. Many have difficulty on account of the shape of the perineum and certain things about the posture. Ordinarily I prefer to examine the way I did here,—by getting my arm between the patient's legs. Some prefer to work with the arm beneath, but I never can work as well that way. If you have the arm between the legs then you have a powerful lever in your elbow to keep the patient from squeezing too hard, but if you have your arm below you have no control, except to beg him not to do that, and with the best intentions in the world, the man may not be able to oblige you. In the case of a male you can have him standing up and leaning over the side of a chair.

A woman is examined in the Sims' position.

Dock reprimanded a student for having failed to make a rectal examination.

DOCK: Have you examined him?

STUDENT: I have not made an internal examination. I did not have the facilities.

DOCK: What facilities?

STUDENT: I didn't have a speculum.

DOCK: The only speculum you need is the speculum you have at the end of your finger. To get the finger greased and soaped and make a simple examination is something everybody should practice and so we will have one person practice it now.

The student reported he felt a strong sphincter, "redundant patches of mucosa hanging down," an enlarged prostate, and internal hemorrhoids. Dock said hemorrhoids "feel like a bunch of earthworms. I remember when I was a kid studying medicine they used to make very good hemorrhoids by filling veins with gore of some kind and bunching them up."

James Arneill had spent the summer of 1901 in Boston, and on return to Ann Arbor he said that all the genitourinary surgeons he saw there used a finger cot for rectal examination. Thereafter the transcript occasionally records that Dock called for a glove or finger cot before doing such an examiantion.

Dock demonstrated the use of a sigmoidoscope. "The battery is out of order, its chronic condition, and we will have to depend on daylight." He said a Kelly proctoscope is much more satisfactory than the previous instrument,[1] and he showed the students how to use it. The instrument is oiled and gently passed all the way in. Dock said:

> By withdrawing it you can see the whole length as you withdraw it. We let these instruments go by their own weight. You never force them because the minute you begin to force them, you lose the sense of touch. In using an instrument like this, the best thing is to let the patient do the work. It is painful and if you push you are likely to increase the difficulty; but if you get the point over the outlet, and get the patient to bear down then you are all right; and you should never take the plug out until you are certain it is in.

Cause and Cure of Hemorrhoids

Dock asked a student.. "What do you gather from the history of his hemorrhoids?" and then Dock gave an impromptu lecture on the subject.

> Is it a common occurrence in his condition? Yes, it is very common. . . . On examining him we found that he has no external hemorrhoids but moderately well developed internal hemorrhoids. The hemorrhoidal veins are large and swollen; there is no ulceration; they are not bleeding now yet they are quite large enough to give him a great deal of pain, especially if he has any difficulty with his defecation. . . . They are probably associated with a condition of the portal circulation, but they occur so often in other conditions that it is worth while thinking about some of the other causes. In general pressure is one of the causes. Constipation is often a cause because it favors congestion of the veins. Diarrhoea is sometimes a cause by setting up an unusual condition of the veins in a different way. Many people believe they are common to people who lead sedentary lives; they have them not because they lead sedentary lives; but because they are likely to be constipated because they are careless about their habits much more so than people of lesser degrees of intelligence. It is interesting to compare the ratio of the disease between classes who lead sedentary and ac-

tive lives; it is rare, for example, among students and common among soldiers. . . . [T]he matter has been worked up with a great deal of care namely, in the German universities. Students there take very little exercise in the ordinary Anglo Saxon way. The soldiers are the same age and exercise from five to sixteen hours a day, practically all the time. . . . [T]hese soldiers ought to be the last people in the world to have hemorrhoids. But the reason is not difficult to see. In many of their exercises they have about 70 lbs. of stuff on their backs that they have to carry, and very often they wear belts or uniforms that constrict them around the abdomen. Of the dietetic conditions that enter into hemorrhoids, the worst is pepper. The fact is quite certain that for most people who have hemorrhoids all sorts of hot spices or seasonings make hemorrhoids worse; pepper, mustard, ginger very often have a very irritating effect so that they can't eat at ordinary hotel or restaurant tables where the food is seasoned to please the rest of the people. In regard to the treatment, there is a great deal of confusion on the subject. Many people propagate the idea that hemorrhoids are always a subject for surgical interference. Many get along perfectly well and can be removed without operation; that is the reason the non-operative advertisers in the papers can afford to keep up their advertisements; but he saves time and trouble by having a radical operation done. [As for treatment]: We simply throw out the causes when we have reason to think it may do some good. The next thing is to regulate the defecation which may be done in a very broad way by attention to diet, habits of eating, stomach, teeth, habits of defecation which can be corrected, and then to the use of the best laxatives to keep regular action, such as Cascara Sagrada which, in my opinion replaces all cathartics recommended. . . . [V]ery often you can get along without that by using morning drinks of cold water. Now if the hemorrhoids are painful and these methods are not rapid enough in their action then there are various things that can be used to improve the condition more rapidly. You can apply ice in the form of the ice bag or ice plasters or hemorrhoid cooler, a metal plug that passes into the opening of the [blank] and kept with ice water or cold water circulating through it.

Dock said witch hazel had been introduced into medicine for treating hemorrhoids. Lauder Brunton recommended its use both externally and internally,[2] but Dock did not see how it could have any effect on the veins when taken internally.

Constipation and Autointoxication

Constipation, Dock said, could be prevented by adding bulk to the diet. In cases of chronic constipation the bowels might be started to move by washing out the stomach. Dock told students not to give cathartics in cases of severe constipation; there is danger of intussusception of the small bowel. Nevertheless, he preferred large doses of calomel, and he said that the dose he used sometimes caused a house officer to faint. When a student recommended castor oil for a baby, Dock asked how he would give it.

> STUDENT: I would give it with a teaspoon.
>
> DOCK: If you tried that the oil, with a vigorous looking child like that, will land on your shirt front. You take a tablespoon, knowing that most will be lost, and you give it in this position; you hold its nose, and the child opens its mouth, and you never let go until the oil is down. The child will hold the oil in its mouth until it has to breathe, then it will breathe and swallow the oil.

When a student said a patient should have massage for her constipation, Dock replied:

> Tell us about that.
>
> STUDENT: The rubbing should be up the right side and then across and down on the left side.
>
> DOCK: Who will do it?
>
> STUDENT: The nurse; or she might do it herself.
>
> DOCK: Can she do it herself? How are you going to get a nurse? Suppose she lives where there is no nurse?
>
> STUDENT: She might use a ball.

DOCK: Yes, you can use a cannon ball, but that after all is not the same as massage. It is a very curious thing that massage as carried out by doctors is so neglected. It is one of the striking peculiarities of practice in this country, as I have pointed out before. A patient who needed massage, in many parts of the world, would get it from the doctor himself who would give it instead of writing a prescription for a cathartic, and make the proper charge. Here a doctor doesn't give it himself for reasons best known to himself, and doesn't have anybody else give it because there is nobody to give it.

When a student presented another constipated patient, Dock said:

Suppose you read her history.

STUDENT (Reading history).

DOCK: You seem to have a very well worked up history and physical examination, and what do you conclude?

STUDENT: Autointoxication from constipation which probably causes neuritis along the intercostal and abdominal nerves.

DOCK: That sounds like a reasonable conclusion, but after all is it satisfactory? How constipated is she?

STUDENT: She has been entirely dependent upon cathartic measures until she came here. Yesterday she had a small natural movement, the first in over a year.

Upon questioning the patient Dock discovered that she had gone no more than two or three days without a stool.

DOCK: She couldn't appear to be a star performer in the constipation line; for example, some people have stools only every two weeks or longer than that. What idea have you about the autointoxication?

STUDENT: I think it is the absorption of the non eliminated poisons from the large intestine in this case.

DOCK: In the first place, we find she has not had very much, and she has overcome what she had by the regular use of medicine. But the question then is, why does not everybody have it who is constipated?

STUDENT: I think it is a difference in susceptibility.

DOCK: Where did you get your knowledge?

STUDENT: In Osler, I gathered that such cases were not uncommon.

DOCK: They are very often talked about and I strongly suspect talked and written about more than they really occur. Probably there is no word more abused at the present time than "autointoxication," and let me warn you to be very careful about how you use such a term out in practice. There is a practical difficulty in calling a disease autointoxication amongst the laity. (To patient): What do you understand by autointoxication?

PATIENT: I don't know a thing about it.

DOCK: I know two very curious instances where doctors had to leave very important families because they said people had autointoxication: one was the case of a highly intelligent woman, a linguist of some parts, who as soon as she heard the doctor pronounce those words had him put out of the house; because she said, auto, self; intoxication, getting intoxicated, hence the word means secret drinking. And it is no use trying to explain for the more you explain the deeper you get.

Appendicitis

C. B. Nancrede, Michigan's professor of surgery, had been a pioneer in the surgical treatment of appendicitis, and there were few patients with appendicitis on Dock's medical service. However, in a symposium on Mackinac Island in the summer of 1900 Dock had to tell physicians how to make the diagnosis.[3] Estimation of leucocytes is important. That does not require complicated apparatus, only a microscope and practical experience in examining the blood. The next year he told the class:

I met a doctor the other day with a very extensive practice who says that he never saw a case of appendicitis, and more than that doesn't believe anybody else ever did. Those things show how experience is fallacious and judgment difficult as Hip. remarked. The fact that anybody in practice can show up a half-dozen diseased appendices in a bottle in a year would not have any effect on such a man.

Sometimes a patient with suspected appendicitis was sent to Dock from the surgical clinic, and sometimes Dock referred a patient to surgery. Once when a patient was sent to him from the outside with a diagnosis of chronic appendicitis, Dock asked whether the patient should be explored.

You will find that doctors and people have different ideas, some looking on an operation as very serious, others not at all, and some in the middle ground. You will find people who think it is not much more difficult than going and taking a drink and others think it is the most serious so that the moment you say a patient has appendicitis everybody will immediately shout no operation must be done. Suppose we think he had appendicitis and we open in the usual position and find nothing wrong there, then we have to go up to the gall bladder; and suppose neither of those things were right, then we would have to cut open the back and explore the kidney. But surgeons don't like to explore unless they know what they are exploring for.

Then Dock discussed what should be done for a patient who really had chronic appendicitis: "If a man was going into the woods two or three days from a doctor, we told him to be explored before he went off. He followed that advice, had a chronic condition, but so far as I know, he never had any trouble after that." And when to operate: "But the principle that has helped me very much is that the minute a patient has so much pain that he needs morphine, then he needs an immediate operation."
Attacks of appendicitis

can be aided in coming on by certain things, like, for example, unusual exertion; people, for example, who do things without being trained for athletic work and especially if they are careless about eating, eating, for example, large quantities of coarse food or indigestible food like peanuts or grapes with seeds. The old idea was that a single grape or peanut would get into the appendix and produce serious consequences; but the danger of that is very slight, as one can readily see in watching the peanut industry. But they get it from eating large quantities of peanuts and riding a wheel to an unusual extent or skating to an unusual extent.

Diarrhea and Examination of the Stool

Dock often passed around stools for students to inspect and to observe consistency, odor, and color. One stool looked like stagnant water with algae growing in it. Others smelled of sour milk or putrid meat. Some contained blood or mucus. Particles that looked like dried leaves really were dried leaves, but Dock could not decide whether they were tea leaves or bits of lettuce or cabbage. Some stools were foamy, indicating fermentation in the intestine, and students must look for foamy stools of soldiers returning from "Porto Rico" or the Philippines with amoebic dysentery or sprue. Inadequately chewed food ferments in the stomach, and fermentation may continue in the intestine of a patient with achlorhydria. Undigested food may be present in the stool of even a healthy person. Dock said:

> Boiled potato is often very hard to digest and will go through even healthy intestines undigested if the action is rapid. It is the same way with banana. The ripe banana is a pretty digestible food. That we can see from the effect of the food; that more people live on bananas than live on breakfast food. But bananas are not digestible because they are not ripe. They may look ripe, but they have been artificially ripened; put in cellars where Italians live, with rotten hay thrown in to keep up a high temperature, and between the emanations from the hay and the Italians they expect the bananas to get ripe. The result is that it is hard to get a banana far from the sea coast that isn't hard to digest. So we find bananas in stools, very frequently large pieces of banana, and it is a very curious thing that they have been mistaken for pieces of worms. A case

UNIVERSITY HOSPITAL

DEPARTMENT OF INTERNAL MEDICINE

STOOL EXAMINATION

Diet ....

MACROSCOPIC CHARACTERS.—Color ......Odor......Reaction......

    Form ....

    Blood ....

        Occult. (Note color changes)........................

        Time of reaction ....

....

    Food Particles ....

    Mucous characters ....

....

    Parasites ....

MICROSCOPIC CHARACTERS.—Blood ....Protozoa........

    Food remains $\left\{\begin{array}{l}\text{muscle fibers,} \\ \text{unaltered starch} \\ \text{cells, et cetera}\end{array}\right\}$ ....

    Oil droplets ....

    Fatty acid crystals and soaps.............................

    Eggs ....Parasites ....

    Yeast cells ....

    Iodin reaction ....

CHEMICAL CHARACTERS.—

    Sublimate test—color ....

    Gas development ....

    Remarks ....

....

....

....

....

....

                Examined by.....................

FIGURE 12. Form used in Dock's department for reporting examination of the stool.

came under my observation several years ago. A specimen was sent to me with the request for the particular worm in it. I wrote back to the doctor, it was from a clinical laboratory run on commercial principles, that I was obliged to say there were no worms there, but pieces of banana. The sequel occurred a good many months afterwards. A patient came to Dr. Nancrede. When I came to inquire more carefully, I found that this was the same patient who had had a diagnosis of intestinal parasites made. When they got my report they paid no attention to the banana part of it. The patient had gone on eating enormous quantities of bananas. This merely illustrates how difficult it is to make people take the steps to see whether they are right. It would have been very easy for them to have put some of the specimen under the microscope to prove whether I was right or not, and to have the patient stop eating bananas to see that the pieces didn't come away any more. Of course the slight on my authority as a diagnostician is simply a part of the trade.

In order to find out what is going on, the patient must be examined from the teeth down. Give him a purgative in order to "know what you are dealing with in the way of intestinal contents; giving calomel, castor oil and a dose of salts. Then you can put him on a milk diet, boiled milk or malted milk and milk and albumin water, or if not milk, albumin water."

Dock showed students how to spread a sample of stool on a glass slide for microscopic examination, and his directions were reinforced by those in James Arneill's book. The sample should be stained for tubercle bacilli. "A considerable proportion of cases of diarrhoea have a diagnosis of tuberculosis of the intestine, or, as it is commonly called, consumption of the bowels. In some cases the diagnosis is made on bacteriological grounds. But it is important to remember that bacilli may be found in the stools that stain like tubercle bacilli that are not the same." Never make the diagnosis of tuberculosis on staining alone.

Amoebas can be found in a fresh stool sample spread on a slide and kept warm. Dock described the size of amoebas and the movements of their pseudopodia. Other cells might be mistaken for amoebas. Dock had found trichomonads, and his identification had been confirmed by Professor McMurrich of anatomy. Other cells may be mistaken for amoebas. Leucocytes may be present in large numbers, but they as well as trichomonads have no diagnostic significance.

Dock said a patient with chronic diarrhea cannot expect to get well quickly. He put one to bed and cleaned her from above with 1/2 ounce of Rochelle salts and from below with two pints of normal salt solution. He gave milk, broth, and tea, but he allowed no milk for a patient whose stool smelled of sour milk. Medicine, he said, did little good, but he gave some patients bismuth and others acetate of lead. Once he attempted to sterilize the alimentary canal with benzylacetylperoxide until the hospital pharmacy ran out of the drug. Dock prescribed silver nitrate in a capsule, but only for a short time. Any good it did would show up at once.

Mucous Colitis

When a student quoted Osler while presenting a patient with mucous colitis, Dock said there are thirty names for the disease, and it is seldom seen at autopsy. Most patients are women, three or four to one, and we find colitis

> associated with all sorts of conditions, endometritis, fibroids, chronic suppurative processes in the (Couldn't understand word), with anything at all in the internal genitals, and further than that in the rectum. Nearly always a patient who has a direct relation between mucous colitis and pelvic disease gets well when the pelvic disease is removed. . . . But there are cases where there is no operable disease.

The patient has cramping pain in the abdomen, very different from indigestion or gastric ulcer, and she knows that within a few minutes to a few hours she will pass mucus. Dock said:

> The discharges are to be looked after very carefully in all these patients. Sometimes there are mere jelly like masses or white glue, or in other cases in a string, and in still other cases complete casts of the bowel itself; many times they are like a tube. In once case I

have in mind the patient was treated for stomach trouble; she was given calomel, and a few days afterward the nurse showed a complete bowel cast, a typical tube. . . . The striking appearance of the mucus always makes people think that there is some dreadful disease in the colon and intestine and especially in people who know something about the comparative anatomy of the intestine. Sometimes they look like skins or tubes; sometimes they are round and circular up to a foot or more in length; in other words, they look exactly like the inside of a sausage casing, and those who have been raised on a farm think they are sloughing out the lining of the intestine. Or sometimes they think it is tuberculosis; they see the skin coming away and think they have some disease as that; or they have heard of consumption of the bowels, and that in turn has very often a marked reflex effect on them. They get these ideas and keep them to themselves and worry about them until they get worse; or what is worse still, they go to somebody who examine[s] carelessly, stains material with acid fuchsin, finds some acid-fast bacilli and gives a report of tb's. Then the patient is still worse off.

A patient with mucous colitis often has a history of maltreatment of the intestines, she has used unusual quantities of a drastic cathartic or large enemas.

For example, we had a young girl here with pelvic disease who could take 4 qts. of enema at one time and get it clear around in the ascending colon. I would not have believed it if we had not seen her demonstrate it, and we could demonstrate over and over again by splashing that she got the whole four quarts inside of her and got it clear over on the right side. That requires a great deal of practice.

When he described a patient whose pain and mucous discharge came on in "storms," Dock said:

Many claim the whole thing is due to (Couldn't hear) secretion of uric acid into the intestine, the reaction being changed, the mucus has a chance to accumulate. In [blank] the secretion is alkaline, and you know that mucus is all soluble in alkali, and so the reason that it does not accumulate is because the alkaline secretion dissolves the mucus. During one of these storms there is a great increase in the uric acid, and consequently the mucus is not dissolved.

Dock said:

One thing in such patients is that they have a general neurosis; sometimes they are victims of psychoses of some kinds; sometimes it is necessary to find whether the patient hasn't gotten on the other side of the border line.

In discussing another patient, he said:

The most important thing undoubtedly is the neuresthenia. The patient constantly thinks of nothing but her "intestines" as she calls them. She can tell you each movement of each individual inch of her intestines just as well as if she had them on a plate. She seems to think of nothing else.

"The neurotic part," Dock said, "usually requires treatment," and he prescribed tincture of nux vomica, beginning with an "ordinary dose" and running up to 40 or 80 drops a day before meals. However:

STUDENT: I would treat her nervousness.

DOCK: How?

STUDENT: I would give her strychnia or nux vomica.

DOCK: Most of these patients are quite irritable enough without giving them strychnia.

A patient should be given as full a diet as she can take.

It is interesting to see that many of them do better if put not on a soft diet such as soft toast or soft boiled eggs, but if we give them harsh vegetables or even some mechanical irritant, e.g. sand along with the food. At any rate a coarse vegetable diet, especially greens, seems to do most of them a great deal of good. . . . Some men go to the extent of using such coarse diet as seeds of all kinds; theoretically that is a very nice thing; but if you put yourself in the patient's place and are fed on seeds of various kinds it is not so very nice. I never heard of a man who recommended this treatment trying it on himself.

Give plenty of water, not less than two quarts a day, to keep the feces moist. See that the patient has regular stool, and the simplest way to do that is to give small enemas, a half pint of cool water. You might even give cascara daily.

Another treatment is an olive oil enema.

It is given probably at night after nine o'clock and given very high, as much as 400 c.c. at a time, and it is better to wash the olive oil in water, and then using quite a few pillows to raise the patient's buttocks and inject the oil as high as possible, and the patient usually keeps it in all night and the next morning the bowels are irrigated with normal salt. The object seems to be this: the bowel is not left empty over night and does not have a chance to contract down and set up irritation by one side being against the other.

Nevertheless, treatment is difficult.

Don't get the idea that all this is to be done at once, but merely that you follow the course of the disease and keep your eyes open, and don't tell the patient that what you give her the first day is going to cure her, or even what you give her the second day.

Worms: Diagnosis

On March 11, 1904, the patient demonstrated was a Philippine veteran who passed as many as twenty-five bloody stools a day.[4] The stools were composed of little pink granules, the size of millet seeds, and students examined them under the microscope. Dock remarked:

You will see bodies that are usually round, granular in appearance, something like a leucocyte, but containing in the center a lot

of greenish things that are the size of blood corpuscles in the preparation. Or you will see a clear object sometimes looking almost
homogeneous or others the color of ground glass. Sometimes you
will see these things move and sometimes the body throws out a
definite lobe. Here they are rather large and vary as a matter of
fact from 15 to 35 microns.

Dock showed blood from a patient with malaria for comparison. "It will
be a good thing for all to see these amoebae. So I will stop the clinic now
and you can look at these preparations."

When the patient was treated with castor oil and enemas of normal
saline containing an antiseptic, eggs of ancylostoma, hookworms,
hatched as far as the embryo stage, were found in his stool. Dock said:

The eggs are so few, and the eggs are in proportion to the number
of worms; and in as much as the eggs come from high up in the abdomen they get uniformly distributed in the faeces, so that if you
examine a certain amount of faeces and count the eggs you get the
number of worms. Now, he has nine eggs or he had four or five
eggs per centimeter. That would indicate that he has not more
than ten worms.

Dock said the worms do not multiply in the body, and those few did not
produce enough toxin to be harmful. When Dock treated the patient
with menthol by mouth and then with Epson salts, eight ancylostoma
appeared in the stool. Dock passed the stool around and said: "If any of
you are so unfortunate as to drop the glass and break it I advise you to
leave town as quickly as possible."

On another occasion Dock passed around a bottle containing a
roundworm. The patient had been operated on for carcinoma of the
stomach. "Saturday night at 10 o'clock the patient vomited and
brought up this beast much to his own comfort because when he saw
that he said that was the cause of his disease and felt sure he would now
get well." Dock said roundworms are not common in Michigan. They
are dangerous when vomited, for they may get into the larynx. They
also get into the bile ducts and gallbladder.

Dock devoted much time to discussing diagnosis and treatment of
tapeworms, for they are "practically the only kind we get in this part of
the world. . . . For those who wish to go into the subject a little further I,

with some hesitancy, might recommend an article of my own in the Loomis and Thompson System that answers by giving a rather bird's eye view of the subject."[5] Dock continued:

Now I want to pass that around and also a lot of other specimens. We have been rounding up some worms lately. Along with that specimen of the egg I will show you the sort of worm that lays those eggs. . . . Here, for example, I have three taenia solium heads, and with the eye lens you can easily see the characteristic shape of the head, and although they are very much shrunken by the hardening they have gone through, yet they give an idea of the extreme minuteness of this body. So it is easy to get lost. . . . The patient may pass an enormous amount of tape worm segments—he passed 40 ft. and that looks very fine—but if the head is not found after careful search then the probabilities are that the worm is still busy or will be very soon. Then one trouble is that people spend time looking for the worm themselves before the doctor has a chance. They stir the material around or pass the stuff through a sieve or do something that involves losing the head, because you can't make people believe how small the head of a tape worm is. You should never leave the inspection to an uninstructed person.

Dock has "measured worms after getting all but the head within a short distance of the neck and then measured them after [he] got the whole thing away, and found that they have grown at the rate of 8" a day."

Often a person with a tapeworm has no symptoms.

In some parts of the country they are so common that one could hardly throw a stone into the street without hitting someone that has one. It is associated with cachexia in which debility and indisposition to work are very important characteristics, and for that reason it has been called the germ of laziness rather wrongfully because not every lazy person has this germ even where it flourishes. . . . Sometimes patients will give you specimens, but they usually come complaining of the symptoms of worms. But the worm phobia is usually a bad condition, and the best thing to do under the circumstances would be to treat the worms.

Worms: Treatment

Dock said:

It is interesting and instructive to follow up the course of treatment under the so-called worm specialists. In the south they are very common, corresponding to the wide existence of tape worms and other parasites of all kinds. Their work, like the work of all quacks, is largely magnified by accidental circumstances that they cultivate to a great extent. Practically all of them are fakers. They don't try to make exact diagnoses. Most of them make a diagnosis by looking into the eye of the patient, which, perhaps, is the best thing to do; for they can tell whether the patient is a willing victim or not by looking into the eye better than if he had a worm by looking in his stool. They give the patient a dose of medicine and then get him into a dark room and have him defecate. The doctor is always there and grabs the vessel as soon as the stool is passed. They go prepared with a sample worm in a convenient bottle and when the critical time comes, show this worm. In fact they don't always have a worm. Gordon told of a quack who carried around the spinal cord from a steer, and of course the spinal cord with the nerve attached had a horrible appearance and people asked no questions and did whatever the practitioner asked. It is interesting to try to find out just how successful their results are; and I have come to the conclusion that they are not more successful than the careful physician who takes careful pain.

Then Dock described how he treated a patient with a tapeworm:

As far as antihelminthics are concerned, some of them are useful, but I have come to the conclusion that male fern is the most reliable of all the remedies and I think it is better to get into the habit of using one thing.[6] Then we give enough to produce the effect, and this means just inside of a dangerous dose. But sometimes they will vomit, and that is a very troublesome thing. In order to lessen the chances of vomiting and make it a little less disagreeable, and help things along one can use shot gun tactics and give the male fern with other things. Put fifteen drops of chloroform in each dose and you can give from fifteen drops up to a dram and then add glycerine and water. If you have a patient that seems to be rather refractory you can add a couple of drops of croton oil. In using it you ordinarily give the patient full catharsis, and from that time on give the patient no food and nothing but a little hot milk and coffee. Then at night you give the patient the first dose of male fern and then along toward morning the worm comes away. You ought to be on hand at this time because if the whole thing doesn't come out entirely, you can very often get it away without losing the head. If the head doesn't come away you have the whole thing to do over again. I have emphasized the necessity of doing the work thoroughly for nothing is so painful as to see a person purged and very often vomiting from the male fern and still not getting the worm away. It makes a bad impression.

Dock called on his early experience:

The Germans who are very successful in this treatment, have a couple of other kinks that they depend upon, and in practicing among German patients I was led to believe there was something in their treatment; for example, they gave herring salad, a very toothsome, but somewhat irritating dish. Another dish is raspberry jam.

Dock said the worms

are very strong, very much attached on sentimental grounds. If they feel any motion on the visible end they hang on in such a way that it is very difficult to dislodge them. You should never try to overcome their strength, but you should hold them by fastening them and tire them out. When you see a parasite partly out the best way is to fasten the worm around a stick of some kind and then give a large injection of warm water or warm saline in the hope that you will surprise it and then be able to get it away.

Once you have the worm

[t]he best way to preserve such a thing for exhibition is the way I have here. I saw it first in the Dresden veterinary school. The

method was devised by Dr. Kochenmeister of Dresden who had a beautiful collection of all kinds of tape worms in the veterinary school in Dresden, one of the most important schools in the world. It is done by spreading out the fresh worm on a pane of glass large enough to put the whole animal on in pieces. You lay the worm over it, putting the sections together. You can't be at all squeamish about the thing. You have to use your fingers, being extremely careful to get you fingers thoroughly sterilized after that because it would be the easiest matter in the world to get thousands of eggs in your system. Then you carefully dry up all the water that runs off from the worm, and in order to have it dry well you should get the water absorbed with cloths or blotting paper. It makes a rather pretty preparation if it be dyed in eosin. Tastes differ, however. Dr. Osborne tells me he prefers a paler pink. While it would hardly do to hang it up in the parlor, it would not be bad for a laboratory or an office.

GALLBLADDER AND
GALLSTONES

10.

IF A PATIENT WERE JAUNDICED,

Dock led the students through a thorough inspection of the eyes and skin to determine the depth and distribution of the pigment. He suggested: "If you look at the patient's hands without looking at the rest of his body you might overlook the fact that he has jaundice. When you press the blood out of his hands you see the yellow color standing out. In the normal hand when you press the blood out you simply get the dull color of the flesh." Sometimes discoloration was not caused by bile pigment. Always ask the patient is he is taking medicines that might discolor the skin. Or:

> STUDENT: He is pale, slightly yellowish tint.
>
> DOCK: It seems he was yellower than he is now.
>
> STUDENT: Well, he has had a bath since then.

A jaundiced patient might say his stools are clay colored, but "It is necessary not only to ask whether the stools have been altered but whether the patient looked to see whether they were altered or not." Dock made the Schmidt test for bilirubin in a stool by rubbing it up with mercuric chloride and looking for green crystals. If the urine were dark, he shook it up to see whether it had a yellow foam. When a dark urine gave no foam, Dock said: "The reason has to do with some very obscure points in physical chemistry that I am far from being able to detail off hand, and that has to do with surface tension." When the sediment was examined, Dock said: "If you look under the microscope you will see cells and casts stained deep yellow, making the examination very easy. That shows the value of always examining the urine." After

178

he had examined a jaundiced adult, Dock had two six-day-old infants brought in. He said:

Here we have something that sounds like a bird's nest. There is no race suicide about this family. Well, judging by the color you might think they were some half-breed race. The have that golden yellow color you see described in the annals of West Indian life that is characteristic of the Creole; but you want to remember, if they belonged to such a race, that at an early age, they would show none of the dark color. Black children are almost as white as white children when they are born; or non-white children at birth are rather ecru or even cream colored. We say they have icterus of the new born. We know it is a harmless condition, although one that sometimes causes a great deal of consternation among the relatives of the subject.

Catarrhal Jaundice

On October 6, 1899, an outpatient from Chelsea, a village a few miles west of Ann Arbor, appeared in the clinic. He was jaundiced but not, as Dock said, so severely as some. His skin was itching, and his urine was dark but not opaque. The patient had nose bleeds, characteristic of jaundice, because "retained bile breaks down the blood."

A week before the patient had eaten chicken salad and ice cream. Vomiting and diarrhea were followed by jaundice. "Now the history of catarrhal jaundice is very clear and of catarrhal gastritis, the jaundice coming on the proper time after." In acute gastritis and duodenitis, Dock said, swelling fills the orifice of the common bile duct and blocks delivery of bile to the small intestine. The prognosis in this instance is good, and the patient's physician is doing the proper thing by treating the patient with a mild cathartic. To control itching, the patient could be given 15 grains of calcium chloride a day and sponge baths of dilute hydrochloric acid, "which has a better local effect on itching than anything else."

This man from Chelsea was the first of many patients with catarrhal jaundice demonstrated in the next nine years. In making the diagnosis

Dock was following the authorities. William Stokes had written of jaundice in 1839: "The third source of the affection is the disease of the mucous surface of the stomach and duodenum, the most important because it is the most frequent cause of jaundice."[1] Virchow had asserted with emphasis: "Für mich steht es fest, dass *Icterus catarrhalis so viel bedeutet, als Katarrh der Portio intestinalis ductus choledochi*."[2] The bile duct is plugged by an epithelial mass rather than by mucus. Osler agreed with Stokes and Virchow when he said that catarrhal jaundice "is probably an extension of gastro-duodenal catarrh" that occludes the bile duct.[3]

Dock said such a patient is manufacturing bile and that it would be better for him if he were not secreting so much.

> DOCK: Here is a man with obstruction of the bile ducts. We want to get the bile running in order to have the benefit of the bile in the intestine and also to prevent damage from stagnation of the bile in the liver and ducts. When we study physiology, what do we learn about the flow of bile?
>
> STUDENT: It is produced by a cholegogue.
>
> DOCK. Name some one.
>
> STUDENT. Bile itself is the best one.
>
> DOCK: Well, that is a popular idea and so you can buy inspissated ox bile in drug stores, but it is after all not a very striking cholegogue. What are the most efficient from a physiological standpoint? Do you know what makes the bile run in the normal individual?
>
> STUDENT. It is caused by the gastric contents being poured out into the intestine.
>
> DOCK: Well, it is partially a chemical stimulation around the outlet of the duct, but still more than that a mechanical stimulation, that is, movement of the intestine, and it is probably from that action that calomel has been given as a cholegogue. However, its effect is not on the liver but on the intestine.

Therefore, stimulate the bowels to move, with phosphates as a cathartic and with cold enemas. Wash out the stomach with warm water.[4] "If it is only catarrhal jaundice then in a few days he ought to show improvement."

The Chelsea man's catarrhal jaundice was the result of gastric upset caused by chicken salad and ice cream. However, Dock recognized that there is another kind of infectious jaundice. "When we say infectious we are more likely to think of epidemic jaundice." Of a patient seen the next year, a boy too young for gallstones or a tumor, Dock said: "You often find out that jaundice of that kind comes in simple small epidemics in single towns or villages, not extending far away, indicating some common source of infection."

Gall Stones

A patient came to the hospital with a history of occasional severe cramping pains. Dock asked the students to suggest a diagnosis, and he commented on their suggestions.

> Gastralgia ("Gastralgia hurts just as much as a stomach ache but it sounds better.")
> Appendicitis
> Intestinal obstruction by a new growth
> Something he has eaten ("Intelligent people find out about this cause and stop.")
> Renal stones ("There are certain cases of renal calculi that have some of the symptoms of gall stone colic, and sometimes these are even associated with jaundice.")

The patient, when questioned by Dock, said he had been yellow after the cramps, but not before his stool was light colored. Dock said the diagnosis was clear and sent the patient immediately to the surgical clinic.

After he had inspected a similar patient, Dock said:

> The next thing is to palpate, and we do that with the object of finding out whether the patient has any pain, and in the second place whether we can feel anything abnormal in the abdomen. We

begin with light palpation, and we go up in the liver region. We are trying to make a direct diagnosis of gall stone colic, but we have to remember that that may be the wrong diagnosis. He might have a gastric ulcer. We try to bring out the tenderness in the epigastrium. We next try to palpate the gall bladder region, remembering that in some cases of gall stone colic, even at intervals, the gall bladder may be enlarged, and we may feel the gall bladder under the right margin of the ribs. Of course, it may be larger, it may extend down the right side. We fail to find it here. We next examine the liver dulness to see if there is any change in that. We find the liver dulness begins on the lower border of the 5th rib and the parasternal line and extends to the margin of the 6th rib, so that the liver cannot be said to be enlarged. At present there is no positive evidence that he has such a condition of the gall bladder.

Dock described how to detect stones in the stool after the patient had been given an enema. Stir the stool thoroughly with dilute carbolic acid, put it in a "Boas sieve," and run water through it. Sometimes a patient himself found the stones.

DOCK: What did they look like?

PATIENT: They were a brownish color on the outside and running through them white streaks like lard.

DOCK: Were they shiny or not shiny?

PATIENT: After they were out 24 hours they were calloused.

DOCK: How big where they?

PATIENT: From a kernel of wheat up to a fair sized bean.

DOCK: How many were there?

PATIENT: Seventeen.

DOCK: Did you keep any of them?

PATIENT: No sir.

Dock thought they might have been fecal matter but more likely pigmented stones. He said that considering the enormous number of persons that have stones, 90% of all women over middle age and almost as many men, stones in the stool are rare. By 1907 Dock had given up looking for them.

In 1906 Dock asked a student what he would do next with a patient suspected of having gallstones.

STUDENT: I'd try the x-ray.

DOCK: That is an important thing, and it is important to understand the position of the x-ray examiantion in such things. When x-rays were first used in diagnosis, of course gall stones were one of the first things experts got at, and all said gall stones would not produce any shadows because there was not enough mineral in the gall stones to cause any obstructions to the ray. However early examinations were made usually from old gall stones and they failed to get anything at all; afterwards it was found by x-raying wet gall stones that they removed at an operation that they would show, and it was demonstrated that they could occasionally be shown in the body. But they still remain very difficult objects to show with a skiagraph. In order to show them it is necessary to have them in a good position. In the next place it is necessary to have a patient who is not too large.

As a last resort, gallstones could be sought at laparotomy. Reuben Peterson, the gynecological surgeon, wrote that during abdominal section for pelvic disease the incision should be large enough to permit palpation of the gallbladder.[5] Dock tried that once when Peterson operated. Dock told his students: "It must be said in my own defense that I am not familiar with wearing rubber gloves, and that made a difference. [The abdominal wound was not very far from the liver], yet when I tried to examine it it seemed as if it was about two feet from the liver."

Dock asked a student what he would do if a patient with jaundice, itching skin and attacks of colicky pain sent for him.

DOCK: What would be the most important thing to do?

STUDENT: Keep her quiet and give her a hypodermic injection of morphine.

DOCK: How much would you give?

STUDENT: Probably 1/2 grain.

DOCK: Would you give it alone or give it with something else?

STUDENT: I don't think I would combine it with anything else.

DOCK: What do you think about that, S******?

SECOND STUDENT. You could combine it with atropine.

DOCK: How much?

SECOND STUDENT: 1/100 grain.

DOCK: What else could you do to relieve her pain?

SECOND STUDENT: You could give her bromides.

DOCK: Hardly.

SECOND STUDENT: You might give her chloroform.

DOCK: Yes, you could chloroform her. It is always better to use morphine and atropine first. Patients have been kept under chloroform for eight days; about half time anaesthesia, the rest of the time going under or coming out. [That they were no better] anybody who understands the pathology of gall stones would be ready to expect, but they would know that if chloroform did any good at all it would do it at once.

Dock gave an injection to a patient who repeatedly complained of pain. "But it is interesting to note that the patient admitted she felt a little better, because it contained as its chief ingredient H$_2$O."

Question of Operation

Dock said that although he was a great friend of exploration of the abdomen, that ought not be done until other methods were exhausted. If the patient has only catarrhal jaundice, he ought to improve in a few days. "Any patient who has jaundice which lasts four months—*I* should say a month—should certainly be explored." What do you tell the patient?

STUDENT: That perhaps he is suffering from neoplasm or stone.

DOCK: You might further say, "At any rate you have an obstruction that has not subsided and if you are not relieved soon your liver, kidneys and blood will suffer from it; so it would be a wise thing to have a laparotomy and have done whatever becomes indicated by the laparotomy." [In practice you might also say]: "The danger of opening and finding out what is the matter is not very great. Any danger that would come, depends on the disease that is there; the worse it is, the more you need the operation early. If there is anything there it might be possible to treat it, and if the condition is too complicated and too far advanced the only thing to do is to close the abdomen."

Once the decision is made to operate:

Then the question is what are you going to do? You will say you can't open up all such patients. But you can open up more than you think. The next thing is, are you going to open up yourself? This is an important point because you can't send all your patients to an experienced surgeon. If you have the facilities for operating, I think such a case would be a good case for even a beginner to take. A young man who has had training in surgical technic and has seen a certain amount of surgical work could say that it would be a good case for a beginner to take. Kehr, the great gall bladder operator, for example, says one should not operate unless he has seen 200 or 300 operations.

Dock was quoting Prof. Dr. Hans Kehr of Halberstadt who, when he reported his own 433 laparotomies for gallstones, wrote:

Deshalb meine ich, dass der Artz solche Operationen ausführen soll, der ganze Zeit diesen Kranken widmen kann und da der practische Artz andere Verpflichten hat, is er selten im Stande, die Nachbehandlung bei einem Gallensteinoperierten so durchzuführen, wie sich das gehört. Den schönen Grundsatz in der Chirurgie: "Nur nicht schaden!" wird der in der Chirurgie nicht besonders ausgebildete Practiker nur dann erfüllen, wenn er die Gallensteinoperation vollständig einem Specialisten, dem Chirurgen überlässt. Man wird mir Egoismus, etc. vorwerfen—ich bin darauf gefasst—aber das kann mich nicht abhalten, meine Meinung offer auszusprechen.[6]

Dock continued:

> That sort of advice, however, seems to me to go right in the face of
> the proper point of view. Very few people can do that. There is an-
> other way to grow. For example, the way Kehr grew was by taking
> such cases. He had not seen anything like 300 when he began.
> There are gall stones one should fight shy of, either send to some-
> body else, or not advise operation at all.

After the operation had been successfully performed by Nancrede, Dock
justified his advice. The operation had been difficult, but they are always difficult, more so if the stone is in the common duct, most if it is in
the hepatic duct. If a beginner found such a condition he could not relieve, he could close up, or he could drain the gallbladder.

> [O]r finally, you can try to finish the operation and have the mis-
> fortune of finishing the patient at the same time. . . . You may, by
> beginning that way, develop into a Kehr or a Mayo. . . . Under-
> stand I am far from advocating recklessness in such a case, but I
> know many that have done well in the hands of competent but un-
> known men.

Not all patients went to surgery. In one patient Dock found a gourd-
shaped mass in the liver and no signs of malignancy. The patient was
likely to have a severe hemorrhage. "That could be told by the coagulability of the blood." At the end of the transcript Dock wrote in pencil:

> Op postponed—pat began to bleed in the skin—Died.

INFECTIOUS DISEASES: TYPHOID FEVER

11.

THROUGHOUT DOCK'S TIME
at Michigan, the medical students had extensive experience in diagnosis and treatment of typhoid fever, and some medical students themselves contracted the disease. Dock and Victor Vaughan, the dean of the medical school, had even more extensive experience. Vaughan, together with Walter Reed and E. O. Shakespeare, had been appointed to a commission to investigate fever in military camps during the Spanish War of 1898. At the commission's request, Dock was made an acting assistant surgeon, and during September 1898 he did autopsies and bacteriological investigations in army camps, demonstrating that typhoid fever, and not malaria or "typho-malarial fever," was the cause of immense morbidity and mortality among the troops.[1]

Typhoid Fever in Michigan

Vaughan began to analyze drinking water from Michigan when his hygienic laboratory in the university's hygiene and physics building was completed in 1888. He found pathogenic organisms in water supplies from more than forty Michigan communities.[2] He repeatedly found typhoid bacilli in Ann Arbor's drinking water, and he traced one Ann Arbor epidemic of fifty-nine cases of typhoid fever to a single milk supply.

There were 2,874 reported cases of typhoid fever in Michigan in 1898 when the state's population was slightly over two million. There were 634 reported deaths for a death rate of 24 per 100 cases. The prevalence of typhoid fever was underestimated because, as the Board of Health said, "Many health officers reported only fatal cases, so that the total number of cases for each year was much in excess of those given." Many cases of typhoid fever were diagnosed as "influenza or malaise," and there is no way of determining the number of undiagnosed cases. Experience at the University Hospital showed that there must have been many. There was no improvement while Dock was in Michigan, for there were 2,656 cases reported in 1908, and the death rate was 27 per 100 cases.[3]

Source of Infection

When Dock presented a woman with typhoid fever to the class, he said that she had probably got it through "contact" with her daughter. He explained that contact is not the same as contagion; contact refers to exposure to excreta and soiled bed clothing and the like. Doctors and nurses in the University Hospital rarely get typhoid fever because they are careful. "Laundry people infect themselves." Dock said some persons believe all transmission of typhoid fever is through contact, but "most cases are still water cases."

A student from Detroit had typhoid fever. Dock remarked:

We look to Detroit water as the cause of infection, probably because there is always typhoid fever there, but even if he wasn't drinking water that might have been infected there, then we have to investigate all the more carefully the other possible sources. Then the question comes up, could he possibly have had the typhoid fever here? What do you think about that? Yes, he might be the first in a series; but in every case where a doctor sees a suspected typhoid it is his duty to find out the local conditions; e.g., last fall in Milan [Michigan], when one or two cases got typhoid it was not remarkable, though it should have led to an examination of the water, and probably did; one or two people might have got it off an excursion; but when cases pile up so that 20 or 30 or 40 people got it, then it became quite clear the infection was there, so they got it either from the milk or the water.

Then Dock described the epidemic investigated by E. O. Shakespeare:

> We look on typhoid fever as an autumnal disease, but some of the most serious epidemics have occurred in the winter time, not in the coldest part, but usually after a heavy thaw. So it was in the town of Plymouth, Pennsylvania, a good many years ago. In those cases the source of infection is easy to trace. In Plymouth a miner was sick living in a house some distance up the creek; the stools were thrown out every day in the snow. A heavy thaw came and all the ice and snow melted, and in about two weeks after this, people who drank water taken indirectly from that creek got typhoid; those who drank the other kind of water—there was another supply in town—did not get it.

Dock wrote that patients in the University Hospital were chiefly students aged eighteen to twenty-five, domestics or housewives, none of "the broken down cases in some city hospitals."[4] Also, he told his class:

> Every fall we have a half a dozen or more cases of typhoid fever with students. They are nearly all treated in town or over here and their excretions go into the river. In the cases of the hospital, we try to disinfect the stools and urine before they are emptied into the sewer. Just how perfectly this is done there is always a certain amount of question. Then the question is, how dangerous is that to people who live down the river. That risk is great, but this is a selfish world; we don't care about those down the river; they just have to look out for themselves. Of course that is all wrong. These things I mention not with the idea of criticizing anybody or any corporation, but simply on account of their general medical importance. People will not ask you to advise them about the location and character of their water supply and pumping stations or anything of that kind now [1907], but the time will come when people take an interest in things of that kind. People will realize, as they have in Europe, that there are better things to do with rivers than to pump all sewage into them and then drink it up again, and when that time comes doctors will have a chance to give people some useful information.

Diagnosis of Typhoid Fever:
Physical Findings

Dock expected his students to see patients first hand, not only on a bed wheeled into the pit. "Students come back here and say that they had better chances here of seeing such cases than in many hospitals where there is more material." Then students would not make the mistake, for example, of diagnosing typhoid fever as "brain fever." To emphasize the importance of seeing the earliest condition, he showed a patient who had just come in after being sick for a week. The patient was anxious and apprehensive, and he was breathing through his mouth. His color was dusky, and his skin looked sodden, as though it were water-soaked. Earlier Dock had said he was shocked to see such ignorance of the typhoid tongue, and he demonstrated that there was a white coat on the middle of the tongue but that the tip was red. Dock had the students look for rose spots on the abdomen. Sometimes the spots were flea bites rather than the characteristic slightly raised, flattened papules. Or as with another patient:

> One interesting thing is that he came in with a diagnosis of typhoid fever. Said he had a "beautiful eruption." Usually the typhoid eruption is so scanty that we do not speak of it as beautiful. One spot might be beautiful, but it seems to me that one could not think this the ordinary way of describing typhoid spots. So, although I heard this without any argument, with the man who made it, I suspected the patient had something other than typhoid. It was rather a measly eruption in more ways than one.

This particular patient had a leucocyte count of 15,000, whereas typhoid patients usually have no leucocytosis. In cases of doubtful diagnosis, Dock said, absence of leucocytosis points to typhoid fever and its presence points to something else, appendicitis for example.

The spleen becomes enlarged early in the course of the disease. Dock said: "I can't imagine anybody with so little enthusiasm as not to see and feel all the things that can be found out there. Get on the other side of the bed and get your hands in the right position and get her to breathe carefully and you will find a spleen you will never forget." But once when Dock found an enlarged spleen, he said: "It doesn't often happen that a person over 50 has a large spleen in typhoid fever."

Tympanites and diarrhea come on in the second week, and Dock passed around in a fruit jar the stool of a typhoid fever patient, "not to be looked upon as an entirely aseptic proceeding." It is a bad sign when the patient becomes incontinent, and if the patient lies in the excreta half an hour she is likely to develop bed sores.

Both Curshmann[5] and Osler[6] had described the "ambulatory form" of typhoid fever in which "the patient keeps about and attempts to do work, or perhaps takes a long journey to his home."

STUDENT: Another physician said he had walking typhoid.

DOCK: Didn't he advise him to go to bed? Do you think it likely that could have happened, that he could be allowed to go about without being sent to bed?

STUDENT: I think so.

DOCK: Yes, we had a man here at one time; he had come in after being told by a doctor he had walking typhoid and should walk all he could and eat all the beef steaks he could. He came in and passed about four quarts of blood by rectum and ended. . . . We could get along just as well if we never heard of walking typhoid fever.

Diagnosis of Typhoid Fever: The Temperature

Every Michigan medical student was expected to know the course of the temperature of a patient with typhoid fever, and in the third year each student was examined on it. On Dock's hospital ward the temperature must be taken accurately and frequently and recorded so that its significance is immediately obvious.

When Dock displayed a charted temperature with a very irregular course, he said:

The probabilities are, first, when you see a thing of that kind, that the temperature is not taken properly. The next thing is to take the temperature correctly. I have found thermometers in patients' mouths and the patient peacefully breathing away with the thermometer there. I don't know what the nurse would have done if she had not been told, probably taken the thermometer out without noticing that the mouth was wide open and marked the temperature where she found it.

Dock said: "Taking a temperature once a day is a clean loss of time. What happens the other 23 hours?" A patient's temperature must be taken every two hours. Dock asked a student to describe the temperature shown on a chart, and the student said that at first the lowest point was in the morning and the highest point about six in the afternoon or a little after. Then the temperature appeared to change; the curve was straight. Dock remarked: "Isn't it rather curious that these lines are all so straight? Isn't it rather unusual for the temperature to follow such a settled course even in young people? How can that be explained? The natural suspicion is that the temperature wasn't taken very often." Dock emphasized this point by displaying two temperature charts. The first showed variations in the patient's temperature in detail. The second had been made by Dr. Cowie by taking only the 6:00 A.M. and 6:00 P.M. readings "in order to show the great difference that may occur in the conception of a case from not having sufficient observations." Dr. Morris had devised a chart with spaces for twelve observations a day and with markings so that what happened in the daytime and nighttime could be seen at a glance.

When he discussed the continuous fever of a patient with typhoid fever, Dock said: "Those are the important things that we want to know in any fever case—the first day he felt bad, the first time he thought he had a fever, the first time he knew he had a fever, and when he took to bed." Because most patients with typhoid fever entered the hospital well along in the course of their disease and without a firm diagnosis, Dock and his students had to use the course of the fever as the most important diagnostic and prognostic aid. Curshmann had described the typical course.[7] The patient's temperature is typically lowest in the morning and highest at midday or evening. In the first week it ascends over three to five days, with the evening temperature 0.6 to 1.0°C higher than that of the previous day, attaining its definitive height by the end of the week. Then the fever is continuous at about 40 to 41°C with diur-

Day of the disease.

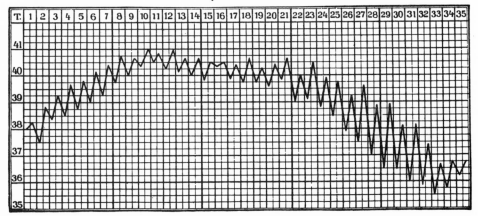

FIGURE 13. Temperature curve of a man of twentyeight with typhoid fever. The attack was severe and somewhat prolonged, but there were no complications. (From H. Curshmann. W. Osler, ed., *Typhoid Fever and Typhus Fever.* Philadelphia: W. B. Saunders and Co., 1902, p. 138)

nal variations of 0.3 to 0.5°. In a third period from the middle of the fourth week, the temperature becomes markedly intermittent or remittent with morning temperatures 1.5 to 2.0° lower than the evening temperature. Finally, the temperature is subnormal for a while. With this knowledge Dock could determine the stage of the disease and know what to expect. For example, a patient entered the hospital with a fever of three weeks' duration and his physician's diagnosis of malaria. Dock soon proved that the patient did not have malaria, pneumonia, peritonitis, or general miliary tuberculosis. He was probably in the fourth week of typhoid fever, and the temperature should begin to descend in a week. A sudden fall during the period of continuous fever heralded a complication, and failure to become subnormal at the end indicated intercurrent sepsis or the probability of a relapse.

Diagnosis of Typhoid Fever: Laboratory Studies

On February 15, 1907, Dock said: "What one thing ought one to think of this time of year? That is influenza, the typhoid form of influenza that resembles typhoid so closely that before the days of the Widal it was difficult to tell them apart."

The Widal test for typhoid fever, used at Michigan throughout the period of the *Clinical Notes*, had been described by Fernand Widal in 1896.[8] Widal mixed serum of blood obtained by venipuncture with a culture of what he called *bacille d'Eberth* and incubated the mixture at 37°C. If the test were positive, the culture tube was clear at the end of twenty-four hours, for "les microbes se précipitant en amas au fond du vase, sous forme de flocons et de pellicules blanchâtres. . . . Formation d'un precipité visible à l'oeile nu, immobilisation, agglomeration et déformation des microbes, tels sont les éléments du phenomène."

Dock did not do venipuncture, and in Ann Arbor the test was made with fingertip blood in a manner somewhat different from that also described by Widal. James Arneill had seen Richard Cabot perform the Widal test in 1901, and Arneill's description of the method in his manual may be paraphrased:

> Draw blood from a finger tip or ear lobe into a small bore glass tube. Seal one end of the tube in a flame, and centrifuge it. Make a file mark at the junction of cells and serum, and break the tube. Blow the serum into a recepticle. Dilute one drop of the serum with ten drops of water, and add one drop of the mixture to a drop of typhoid culture. Examine under a microscope. Add ten more drops of water to the first dilution of serum for a 1:20 dilution, and so on. Or dilute serum in a white blood cell counter. Don't use dried blood, because it is impossible to tell the dilution.[9]

It is necessary to have a lively, motile culture of typhoid bacilli, and in a positive test the bacteria become immobile and agglutinate. "Les amas sont visible sous le champ du microscope quelques instants apres le mélange."

Dock said that "in order to draw diagnostic conclusions from it one must be able to get clumping with a considerable dilution of the blood and the dilution generally agreed upon is 1:40." He said a positive Widal test is usually present from the second or third week, but a negative reaction, though rare, does not rule out the diagnosis of typhoid fever.

Dock maintained his own cultures of typhoid bacilli, but the physician in private practice may have trouble with the Widal test. Dock said: "Very often he can't use the test because he has no laboratory at his disposal or his culture is not taken care of properly and so when he wants the reaction he can't use it; or he sends his material to a city laboratory and experience shows that about three-fourths of the diagnoses are wrong."

On a few occasions an attempt to grow typhoid bacilli from a patient's blood is mentioned in the *Notes*. Once the incubator froze when the gas was turned off, and the next day its temperature rose to 50°C, killing the culture.

The second laboratory test was a version of the diazo reaction introduced by Ehrlich in 1883[10] and modified by innumerable others, including Aldred Scott Warthin. Osler gave a recipe:

A saturated solution of sulphanilic acid in dilute hydrochloric acid and a 0.5% solution of sodium nitrite are kept in separate bottles. At the time the test is made 1 cc of sodium nitrite solution is added to 40 cc of the sulphanilic acid solution, and a few cc of the mixture is added to an equal volume of urine and thoroughly shaken. Then 1 cc of ammonia is allowed to flow down the side of the tube, forming a colorless zone above the yellow urine. If the reaction is positive, a deep brownish-red ring will form at the junction of the two solutions.[11]

Osler found the reaction to be positive in 894 of 1,467 cases of typhoid fever. Osler and Dock as well as Ehrlich found the diazo reaction to be positive in other febrile diseases, tuberculosis and malaria among them, and although Dock or the students often performed the diazo test, one gets the impression that no one gave it much weight.

Treatment of Typhoid Fever: Tubbing

Dock insisted that his typhoid fever patients be tubbed, but he never gave any reasons. Osler listed the good effects: the delerium is lessened, the fever may be reduced though that is not the most important, the heart rate usually falls, bronchitis is benefited, there is less chance of passive congestion of the lungs, and the liability to bed sores is diminished. The strongest reason is that tubbing reduces mortality. At the Brisbane Hospital typhoid fever mortality was 14.8% before and 7.5% after tubbing was introduced, and the experience at the Johns Hopkins Hospital was similar. In a general hospital six to eight typhoid fever patients in a hundred are saved by tubbing.[12]

Dock's enthusiasm for tubbing was expressed in his orders to students:

> I would like to remark too that we have a typhoid patient here who is being tubbed and who will probably need tubbing for some time. I would rather have volunteers for the work. We have a number of sick nurses so that it is rather hard to get nurses to tub the man. I would like to point out that these assignments go. When you are told to tub a man it means that you will tub him or there will be some delay in your graduation.

At another time a student had missed his assignment.

> I would like to remark that while sickness excuses a man from that sort of thing, nothing else does. Buying a heifer or marrying a wife or any minor reason will not go. These tubs are not given to you as punishment, but as a privilege, but a good many of you don't seem to appreciate that fact.

Dock divided the class into detachments and assigned responsibilities. Later he changed the system so that a man was no longer on duty for twenty-four hours; he was required to give only two baths so that he lost only four hours.

A tub held enough water to cover the patient to his neck, and the water was changed every twenty-four hours. A nurse brought the water to the proper temperature by adding hot or cold water. For the first bath, water at 80 to 85°F was used, and it was reduced 5° at a time until 65 or 70°F was reached. The patient was bathed every two hours, and "it does no harm to drop a patient with a fever of 104° into a bath at 70° and keep him there for 15 minutes" while he turned blue and shivered. Dock informed the students: "Quietly proceed without seeming haste. Put a towel about his head, and from a pitcher containing ice water pour over his head very gently a quart at a time. Do it every three or four minutes throughout the bath. . . . Never leave a patient alone in a tub."

Just before the Christmas vacation of 1899 Dock said a woman of twenty-six was "a proper patient to be treated with a cold bath. . . . Now any woman intending to stay over the Holidays will get a good opportunity to bathe the patient. Any junior women can have this opportunity also. Now when you go to bathe the patient don't simply turn yourself into a bathing assistant and think that is all you can do." Observe the patient's tongue, abdomen and spleen. "Anyone with eyes and even a rudimentary cortex can't spend fifteen minutes with a typhoid patient without learning something." Pour water over her head while she wears a rubber cap. It is often worth time and trouble to clip the hair. But "[i]f the patient has not very much hair or if getting the hair wet will not be too much trouble for the nurse, then the hair may be allowed to stay on, especially in the case of a woman who might find some difficulty in getting a wig to cover her hair afterwards."

A woman patient objected piteously to being tubbed, despite Dock's assurance that most patients do not think it painful and do not complain. When he was told of another patient who did not like the baths, he said: "We don't pay any attention to that because it is not unusual. . . . While you should never be afraid to make a patient uncomfortable if it is for his own good, yet if it doesn't do any good, don't do it."

Dock rebuked students who did not observe the patient while bathing him:

Not the least important of all is the fact that people will waste their time trying to bathe a man without seeing him. I would prefer that students if they are too busy to look at the man not look at him at all. Probably the patient would not get along so well, but the damage you do to your own mind by working on a patient without looking at him, is more than the harm done the patient by not being tubbed at all.

Otherwise, tubbing could be done in the dark or by a nurse while the student sat and read a book.

When the patient is in the tub, his skin must be rubbed to bring blood to the surface. Do not rub too hard. "Sometimes I have found a football player rubbing patients so that they rubbed the hair out of the hair follicles." Small abscesses develop in hair follicles when the skin is rubbed too hard.

Tubbing gave the nurse time to put the patient's bed in order. Dock said, "that has always been a problem with typhoid fever. Formerly, the nurse who could not make a bed successfully under the patient, under the covers, moving him gently to the half that was made and slipping the soiled linen out, was not considered as knowing her business." Then the patient was put back in bed without night clothes, for a typhoid fever patient always remained naked under the covers. He was dried with a sheet, and the wet sheet was replaced with blankets and hot water bottles. He waited for the next tubbing in a little over an hour and a half. Some patients were tubbed fifty or a hundred times.

Other Treatment

Once Dock's bacterial culture went bad, and he had to wait for another before he could make the Widal test. He said the patient should be treated for typhoid fever, the more likely condition, for that treatment was as good as any. If she had typhoid fever she would get well; if she had miliary tuberculosis, she would not. When the diagnosis of typhoid fever was certain, Dock gave no antipyretics. He said:

> So our patients are treated, not by medicines that have a very severe effect on them, but by medicines as mild as possible. Suppose, for example, we gave every patient with typhoid fever an antipyretic. That from one point of view would be very instructive; but you might give antipyrin until you are old and gray and not see fever patients but patients with fever plus antipyrin.

If a patient had tympanites, Dock first gave a cool enema or perhaps one containing castor oil and tincture of asafetida. When that failed:

> Didn't you know what we gave him? We gave him turpentine. His tympanites were severe; tongue dry and very tremulous and he looked as if he was going to cry every minute; his whole appearance was that of the typhoid state. So we gave him turpentine

for empirical reasons. Turpentine is an old remedy for typhoid fever and was especially celebrated in this country by Drs. Wood, George G. and Horatio C., his nephew, who looked on it as especially good in typhoid cases that had the typhoid state.

The dose was 10 drops in milk; the danger was nephritis. Dock's faith in strychnine lasted to the end, for describing the treatment of typhoid fever in the University Hospital he wrote in 1908: "Strychnine was used for its supposed stimulating action. When we began to use the blood pressure apparatus we discovered that the stimulating effect could not be measured in the arteries, but we have continued to use it as before."[13]

Diet

The danger of intestinal perforation in typhoid fever was met by diet. In March 1902 the temperature curve of a young man, perhaps a university student, showed that he was recovering satisfactorily from typhoid, and Dock told the class how he was being fed.

> DOCK: Let us read exactly what he is getting. It is very instructive to read actual diet lists. That is probably the greatest need that the young practitioner feels, to know what to give the patient. On the 13th, the patient got 1000 c.c. milk, 400 c.c. broth, 400 c.c. lemonade, 200 c.c. albumin water, 600 c.c. water, and one soft egg.
>
> STUDENT: That is a large amount of fluid.
>
> DOCK: Well, is it a large amount? That is 2600 c.c. plus one egg. But that day he passed 2100 c.c of urine, so that really he was losing weight at that time, if he was passing within 400 c.c. of what he took in. He might easily have lost 400 c.c. by the lungs besides what he lost by his bowels with the use of an enema.

The patient should be given enough water to keep his daily urine volume above 1,500 c.c. Dock continued:

> The next day, yesterday, he got 1200 c.c. milk, one egg, some milk toast, some custard and some rice. By this time it would be quite

safe to give the patient some soft meat. Nearly always begin with fish, if it is convenient to get some good fresh, soft fish, and give it to him in the shape of boiled fish, not fried, or we might even give the patient such things as soft white meat of chicken. Usually we begin with such things rather than red meat, although I know of no good reason for not giving them red meat. It is rather a matter of custom. Then we go on to beef steak or mutton, usually beef steak is a little easier digested. About this time we give him baked potato, well mashed up.

Dock said that milk is really not a liquid but a solid or semisolid food. One can make the curds come down by adding vegetable juice, rice water, Vichy water, or Carlsbad water. Albumin water, he told the class, is made by simply beating up the white of an egg in water and flavoring it with lemon juice. Ice cream could be added to the diet, simply frozen cream with flavoring in it, and so could jelly or thoroughly boiled rice or thoroughly cooked macaroni, of course without any cheese. Meat should be the softest obtainable, sweetbreads or the soft part of oysters.

A few days later the patient had passed the time when he might have perforation, and Dock discharged him: "So inasmuch as convalescence is nearly always more rapid in comfortable quarters he has been allowed to go to his room where he will be seen every day by Mr. Jump [the student] who is familiar with his case so far."

Dock did not mention the hospital kitchen then or on similar occasions, but the dieticians and cooks were clearly up to their job.

Complications and Their Treatment

Perforation of the intestine and hemorrhage were the chief complications. Dock remarked:

So we do all we can to keep up the patient's strength and to keep him comfortable and don't wait until a symptom appears and then fire in some medicine; but knowing certain things that will be liable to develop we do not wait until they develop before doing anything. For example, we do not sit around and wait until he gets peritonitis, but we watch carefully to detect the earliest symptoms of a perforation; so, too, we do not wait until he has a large hemorrhage, I hope; but watch the thing to tell whether he has it long before it is evident on the outside.

Before 1903 blood in the stool was the surest sign of hemorrhage, but many patients, including some who died, had no blood there or less than a half ounce. Hemorrhage or perforation was signaled by a sudden drop in temperature, and this is the reason Dock insisted that the patient's temperature be taken frequently. Once, for example, a patient with typhoid fever had a continuous temperature just below 104°F. A small quantity of blood appeared in his stool. Then his temperature abruptly fell to 96°; a large quantity of blood appeared; and his blood hemoglobin concentration fell to 60 to 65%. This patient was treated with opium and acetate of lead. The hemorrhage stopped, the temperature rose, but Dock said there was still danger of thrombosis, phlebitis, or another hemorrhage.

The sixth edition of Osler's textbook said: "The recent introduction of clinical instruments for measuring blood-pressure has been most useful. (Consult the work of T. Janeway on Blood-Pressure, 1904.)"[14] In typhoid fever, Osler said, the systolic blood pressure measured by Riva-Rocci's method is usually 115 to 125 mm Hg, and the diastolic pressure averages 85 to 100 mm Hg. On October 20, 1903, Dock reported to the class that a patient who had been sick two weeks before he was brought to the hospital had had a sudden drop in temperature. "He might have a hemorrhage that would not show externally for many hours after, but it also shows in the blood pressure by signs that are not well known." If there is another drop in temperature, the patient will become a surgical case. The patient recovered; his temperature rose again; and although there was some blood in his stool he had no other serious symptoms. But at noon on October 27 his temperature fell to 98.6°F, and he was delerious. It is important, Dock said, to take his blood pressure again. As Dock was discussing the patient, he said: "If Dr. Alexander[15] finds anything in the blood pressure, we will hear about it. (Dr. Alexander comes in.) His blood pressure is all right, 130, so we won't send him to the surgeons yet." The patient went home on November 23, for it is safe to send a patient home a week after his temperature is normal.

Dock described another patient whose temperature was falling and who had a great deal of pain: "He has a nervous anxious look, as one might suppose from a senior medical student with the symptoms he had. He thinks of a distinct disease and he is right to think about it, and grows more and more nervous about the conditions." He should be referred to surgery, for an operation should be done before peritonitis sets in. "Quick resort to exploration may do an immense amount of good in case of perforation."

Three months later the student was back at work, and Dock blamed himself for not preventing that. Typhoid fever patients should not do any work for a long time, but with students there is a great temptation to return. Six weeks after he was discharged, the student had a new set of symptoms: fever, chills, a peculiar kind of pain, and a rigid back. This is a "typhoid spine," and Dr. Herdman, the neurologist, diagnosed multiple neuritis. The student did graduate with his class, and he lived to practice medicine in Albion, Michigan, for more than fifty years.

Once Dock told the class about an emergency that had arisen the day before. There had been an abrupt fall in the temperature of a patient with typhoid fever, and there was pain in his abdomen. "The only new sign about the abdomen was the gurgling that has always been present before was absent. The absence of gurgling is a symptom sometimes of great importance and one should always suspect that something has happened to the wall of the intestine to interfere with peristalsis." Dock had sought the advice of the surgeons. That night Dr. Nancrede found rigidity of abdominal muscles and thought the patient was probably getting a perforation. The leucocyte count was 12,000, and the temperature was 104.5°F. Nancrede cited the statistics of his former Philadelphia colleague, Dr. W. W. Keen, that it is better to operate in the second twelve hours than in the first twelve hours. The patient was prepared for operation at one o'clock at night and was operated upon in the morning in the presence of students. Dock said the operation was a comparatively new one. Dock described the condition Nancrede had found: a perforated, inflamed Peyer's patch.

In order to close that the intestine had to be drawn together in such a way that the natural lumen was narrowed down. You must remember that in doing that the swollen Peyer's patch had to be pushed in. [Dock drew a diagram]: Of course, to make an end-to-end anastomosis prolongs the operation, so that it is considered better to cover up the perforation rather than to make a more formidable operation.

The lumen would remain obstructed until the patch sloughed off. About one-fourth of such patients are likely to recover; of the other three-fourths, the condition is hopeless anyway. This patient did recover; his temperature came down; his mind cleared; and his bowels began to move.

There were competent surgeons in the University Hospital, but there might not be one outside. Dock remarked: "If you are not operating yourself the patient and the family should be warned about the necessity of quick operation; sterilized water, room, and everything else should be got ready. Then if you are not operating you should have a surgeon ready to do so." But you must ask whether an operation would be useful: "But in private practice it not only prejudices the person who recommended to operation, but prejudices the operation itself; for if the result is not good then in future cases in the same neighborhood if there is one with particularly favorable indications to operate for signs of perforation, nobody would be willing to operate on account of previous failure."

There might be other complications. The temperature of a patient in the twenty-ninth or thirtieth day of typhoid fever had not gone down as expected, and his ear drum ruptured. Dock thought that it should have been punctured, and he told the students they should learn the technique in case no ear man were available.

I have never seen anyone hurt by a proper puncture. It is better to have that come out than to break. Those very often go on to mastoid complications. In some years it is much commoner than others; but always in measles, scarlet fever, pneumonia and typhoid and very often influenza, the tendency is to have that come on without any symptoms, and you should be prepared to do the work yourself. . . . One disadvantage of having such a satisfactory ear clinic is that we leave these matters to the ear clinic too much.

In ordinary practice one would have to look after that himself, and I would strongly urge all of you to get all you can out of the ear clinic about the complications in acute disease.

Typhoid fever patients died, and a few went to autopsy. A student thought one patient would have died anyway; he had peritonitis, bronchopneumonia, and beginning endocarditis as well as typhoid fever. Dock added two other serious symptoms from the beginning: delerium and tympanites. Dock's description of autopsy findings occupies fourteen pages of transcript, and when he had finished he said: "In a case of this kind a great deal can be done by going over things. Ordinarily we don't cry over spilt milk; but it is always well when we lost a patient to go over the points in the history and find out just where we can improve or sometimes that it is not possible to improve."

INFECTIOUS DISEASES:
TUBERCULOSIS

12.

DOCK INSISTED THAT
his students learn the early diagnosis of tuberculosis. When he discussed the midyear examinations, he said:

> Nearly everybody started off on a beautiful description of an advanced case of tuberculosis, with cavities, night sweats, emaciation, etc. And that is just the trouble, what we need at the present time is a lot of doctors who are able to detect the signs before cavity formation, before sputum begins to form, certainly before night sweats and great emaciation, even before percussion signs come on. It would be worth while for most of you to carefully study all you can about the early symptoms of tuberculosis of the lungs.

A patient in the early stages of the disease might be successfully treated, but there is little or no hope for a patient in the advanced stages. The trouble is that many of the patients who come to the University Hospital with advanced tuberculosis have not been diagnosed early enough. Dock said:

> The patient has the disease that has been known so long and has been worked up so thoroughly that we are better informed about diagnosing it than we are of any other disease, and yet it is a fact that patients having this disease go about without having the diagnosis made for them. That comes from the fact that the physicians that the patients consult do not take the trouble to find out about the disease. They do not find out about it simply because they do not get to the patient. In the first place they do not strip

the patient, and not stripping the patient they do not get the physical signs of lacking expansion over one apex. . . . It is interesting to note about this patient that although she gives this history she came down here, sent down by a doctor who said that he never examined her and did not know what she had. It is a curious thing that she came here for a disease that could have been made known several years ago.

In about one-third of the tuberculous patients admitted to Dock's clinical service, the diagnosis of malaria had been made at some time. Arneill said:

Anyone connected with a hospital where exact diagnosis is made is aware that many times diagnosis of malaria is made where the physician should have made the diagnosis of tuberculosis. So many physicians make the diagnosis of malaria if the patient tells them they have a chill and probably do not strip the patient, fail to examine the chest; and if they did they might not get the sounds of beginning tuberculosis, as it is sometimes difficult.

In another instance a patient had been in bed for eleven months with "la grippe." Dock thought it absurd to be in bed so long with that disease. As an aside, he told the class that grip was not recognized as such eighteen years ago; in those days there was acute cold, tonsilitis, bronchitis or pharyngitis, but no grip. Many experienced persons including Laënnec thought that repeated colds protect against tuberculosis.

In February 1904 Dock "tried to work out the diagnosis that had been made in [three] tuberculosis cases before they came here." One had been treated for liver disease, and another had been treated by an osteopath. The diagnosis had not been made in the third because for two years the patient's sputum had been reported negative. Dock said: "You have only to look at the patients' chest to realize that they have tuberculosis. Then you diagnose in about two minutes by the microscope."

Once the diagnosis is made, the patient must accept it. Dock said:

The patient is one of a kind that we very frequently see in practice. She has symptoms that frighten a great many people very easily.

The minute the patient begins to cough and expectorate they begin to be very much frightened, but she consistently refuses to believe that she has anything the matter with her at least in the lungs. It is very important to try to get such a patient to realize what the condition is, and it is not an easy thing to do. She must understand that steady, persistent treatment is necessary, not medicine.

The Adjective

Dock asked a student who had used the word *tubercular* to distinguish between *tubercular* and *tuberculous*. When she had trouble, Dock said:

The difference is that in the first place very many careful instructors don't make any distinction. They mix things up, but there is a tendency on the part of still more careful people to use "tuberculous" in connection with tuberculosis, so hip joint disease would probably be tuberculous; whereas they use the word "tubercular" in connection with anatomical patterns known as tubercles. We could speak of change in a tubercular process using the word without any reference to etiological meaning; but if we had a process of miliary gummata we could say that was a tubercular process in the lung. Try to get the more etiological term. Don't use tubercular for tuberculous in any form.

Prevalence and Source of Infection

Dock had good reason to insist that his students learn about tuberculosis. In 1898 there were 2,728 reported deaths from tuberculosis in Michigan, and the death rate was 114.2 per 100,000.[1] In Dock's time, improvement was slight, for in 1908 there were 2,512 reported deaths with a death rate of 95.2 per 100,000. Tuberculosis was a young person's disease, for in 1903–1907 the age of death as a perceptage of all deaths was

15–24 years	27.1%
25–34	25.8
35–44	16.6
45–54	9.4
55–64	5.1
65 and over	1.5

Dock cautioned his students not to believe that infants and old persons cannot get tuberculosis.

When a student read the history of a tuberculous patient, it usually said that close relatives had died of tuberculosis. Dock frequently said that "the family history has no bearing on it whatsoever, except as a matter of interest."

Very often people may have tuberculous relatives and yet not be exposed to real danger of infection; with men especially, it is usually more likely that they get their infection at their work. They are in danger of infection from some other workmen rather than from a relative at home whom they may see only a short time every day or not so often as that, by inhaling sputum or getting on their hands or mouth or anything of that kind.

The patients on Dock's service were farmers, lumbermen, and others living in the country or small towns, and Dock used one hundred such patients for an etiological study of tuberculosis in country people. Tuberculosis, he wrote, is not hereditary, and the assumption that it is may be deceptive. "A patient is told that he has "bronchitis" or "malaria," or what not, and assured there is no danger "because there is no consumption in the family."[2]

Dock found no tuberculosis in the parents of seventy-four tuberculous patients, and he pointed out that the proportion was precisely the same as that in the Johns Hopkins Hospital, which dealt with an urban rather than with a rural population. He said:

Many who examine our figures will make much of the fact, that of 100 cases of tuberculosis, one-fourth had a tuberculous family history. To us it seems much more important to know that out of 100 cases three-fourths had no such history. . . . We look upon tuberculosis today not as a diseased inheritance but rather a disease of contagion and we look to the people the individual was most exposed to to find the source of the disease.[3]

Infection, Dock argued, occurred through intimate contact of one person with a tuberculous patient, and he cited case histories and the experiments of others to support his argument. Contact accounted for the fact that in the twenty-six tuberculous families

> 14 exhibit *tuberculosis in other members of the present generation*; namely, 17 sisters and 6 brothers of patients. Of these 23, 13 came from 8 families with tuberculous mothers. . . . [T]hey show a greater tendency of tuberculosis in families with tuberculous parents; greater morbidity of the daughters. . . . [T]he relatively large number of tuberculous children below the age of 25 years may be explained more readily by the greater exposure of young people to infection present in the parents than by prolonged latency of inherited germs.[4]

As for the supposed virtues of rural life:

> The open-air life on the farm and elsewhere is supposed to make infection unlikely. On the other hand, observation among such cases shows how easy infection may be. The long hours of idleness in winter; the habit of using a common living-room, which is often the dining-room, and often overheated, while the other rooms are cold; the carelessness with sputum, often shown by a common use of handkerchiefs, cups, etc.—these far offset any advantage of air and nutritious food.[5]

The Tuberculosis Club

One December Dock said:

> I think it would be a good thing if we had a sort of tuberculosis club, and called on the people who had such cases along about the

beginning of the second semester—no, not at the beginning, that would be too much of a strain—but, say, before the spring vacation, for the combined effort on the treatment of tuberculosis. You can get together and divide up the subject in any way you see fit. . . . Every person who has a tuberculosis case is a member of the Tuberculosis Club and there are no initiation fees and no dues.

The next April eight students reported on

> Early Signs of Pulmonary Tuberculosis
>
> Cough in Pulmonary Tuberculosis
>
> Fever in Pulmonary Tuberculosis
>
> Tuberculin in Pulmonary Tuberculosis
>
> Some Important Complications of Pulmonary Tuberculosis
>
> Treatment of Pulmonary Tuberculosis in Sanatoria
>
> Home Treatment of Tuberculosis
>
> Dietetic Treatment of Tuberculosis.

Dock's comments occupy seven pages of transcript, and he concluded by saying: "I am sure you must all have enjoyed hearing these and there is a great deal of useful information in them. I think we can profitably spend the first part of the next hour in hearing the remaining papers." Those were on

> Tuberculin as a Therapeutic in Tuberculosis
>
> Symptomatic Treatment of Tuberculosis.

Dock said all papers showed a high degree of excellence, and he encouraged the formation of a tuberculosis club in other years.

Diagnosis of Tuberculosis: History and Hemoptysis

When a student presented the history of a patient with tuberculosis, Dock said:

Well, that is a good history. There is a lot of work on it. I see you realize that too, probably. Some teachers never like to assign tuberculosis cases to students because there is too much work on them. For my part, I don't object sometimes to giving other people work to do. I think it is rather an advantage to the student to have a difficult case occasionally, especially in the history taking.

Emaciation is an important sign. A student said:

She comes to the hospital because of loss of flesh and overwork. No more definite statement can be obtained.

DOCK: Is that important? That is one of the most important statements that we can get if the individual can be relied upon. Loss of weight is a certain evidence that the patient is not right.

A woman whose brother and two sisters had died of tuberculosis had a history of pleurisy. Dock remarked:

In many cases the menstrual history is important, but in all serious diseases and those that affect nutrition and in tuberculosis one should enquire about the menstruation. (Reading history): She hasn't been feeling well and worked hard decorating a church. (To students): Of all places of resort churches are the most dangerous. They are not well heated and as she was decorating she went probably there when the church was cold. The ventilation is always poor; the atmosphere is likely to pick up anything about, and usually the heat is furnished from registers in the floor so that the auditors can be properly warmed as they come up the aisles.

Chills and night sweats are also important, and so is hemoptysis. A law student who came to the hospital in November had two spells of spitting blood the previous August and September, "Yet the interesting thing is that the family physician examining him just before college opened thought he could come here." On another occasion Dock asked a student to describe what he saw in a basin.

STUDENT: A central blood clot with white masses mixed in it.
DOCK: What else?

STUDENT: Fluid.

DOCK: What is the most important thing in it?

STUDENT: It is arterial.

DOCK: Are you sure?

STUDENT: If it is very recent—

DOCK: Well, is that so? Suppose you let blood from a vein. Does it always stay dark? What do you think, Barnett?

STUDENT: There was a slight amount of froth.

DOCK: Was it a slight amount? It was quite frothy. That would make you think—

STUDENT: That it came from the lungs.

DOCK: Well, it did come from the lungs of a man just as he was waiting outside. Suppose the patient had a pulmonary hemorrhage, what would you do for him?

STUDENT: I would keep him at rest.

DOCK: How would you do that?

STUDENT: I would avoid all possible conditions of excitement.

DOCK: Would you examine him now? Would you examine him at all? Suppose you were called to a house where a man was bleeding that way and knew nothing about him, would you examine him at all? Well, I think you might examine him a little this way —without disturbing him at all, tell him to breathe quietly and auscult him in order to find out whether he didn't have some disease and you could get an idea of the extent of the disease, but never make him take a deep breath and never make him cough and never percuss him. The patient has not bled any more and the probabilities are that the vessel has been closed. Suppose he was still bleeding, what would you do for him?

STUDENT: You might put an ice bag over the chest.

DOCK (to patient): You have had a hemorrhage before? You are not frightened then? (To students): You see the patient looks very much unconcerned. He has a natural horror of blood if it is his first time. This patient doesn't look as if anything at all dangerous has happened to him, and, of that kind is not particularly dangerous at first; but where the patient is frightened you can give him morphine and to stop the bleeding give him acetate of lead.

Diagnosis of Tuberculosis: The Temperature

Dock said that when he began he had known only hectic fever. To instruct his students he once reviewed the temperature charts of sixty tuberculous patients.

> [Thirty] were intermittent; 12 were remittent, and 10 had no temperature, and in only one there was what might be called continued fever.[6] . . . In pulmonary tuberculosis, we have at times no fever; we have also continuous fever, remittent fever, intermittent fever, and periods when the temperature is below normal. Continuous fever is much like the continuous fever of acute infectious diseases except that the temperature still does fluctuate to a considerable extent; remittent fever reaches a high point somewhere in the afternoon or evening and in the morning descends, but does not reach the normal temperature; intermittent fever reaches a peak during the afternoon or evening as a rule and descends to normal or in some cases sub normal. . . . In summing up then, a patient with a high remittent fever has an unfavorable prognosis. Of course in giving this, I am rather emphasizing fever more than really should be done. A continuous fever is always unfavorable. Intermittent fever may be unfavorable or it may not be. Sub normal and collapse temperature are unfavorable. A temperature of 97 is a sign of weakness as a rule, weakness and often of collapse, a failure on the part of the organism to react against injurious changes.

Fever, Dock said, is important because it is an index to the general treatment of the disease, and consequently "We do not rely much upon the antipyretics."

Diagnosis of Tuberculosis: Physical Findings

A patient had very striking clubbing of the fingers: curved nails and thickening of the phalanx. Dock said:

Whenever you see clubbed fingers it is safe to say that the patient has severe disease of the thorax requiring extensive treatment. . . . [F]rom the days of Hippocrates down they all describe clubbed fingers as part of the picture. . . . The popular idea just at present [1899] is that it is due to a toxin forming in the lungs that affects the hands, especially the extremities, in a trophic manner.

A student described a patient: "On inspection there is not much except that the face is flushed characteristically, and it is not so much as it was two days ago. Inspection of the thorax shows that it is a characteristic long chest, with slight lagging on the left side." The supraclavicular spaces on the left were lower than on the right. Breathing was largely abdominal, and Dock agreed that

[t]he expansion is less and rather lagging in the middle line. We will find out all about it when we get the saddle tape. We fasten these in the middle line, get them even, and we hold them in the middle in front. We find that they stand, on the right side on quiet breathing, at 14 1/4, on the left side at 13. On deep breathing it reaches 14 3/4 on the right side, 13 1/4 on the left. So we find out not only that the right side is larger than the left but the expansion is also less on the left.

Dock asked the students to observe elevations of the skin where he had percussed the chest. This is myodema. "No less a person than Lawson Tait thought it is one of the best signs of tuberculosis. That however is wrong."

A student said palpation revealed tactile fremitus over the right apex and right upper side; there is a cavity in the right apex. In answer to Dock's question, he replied: "Because the note is tympanitic; you get Wintrich's sign with the mouth open, and with the mouth shut a change in the note. You get very distinct moist rales, blowing breathing also on this side." Dock said:

There is no diagnostic sound about a cavity, but there is a certain feature about a sound that we call cavernous that is hard to describe but easy to understand. Where we talk over the mouth of a bottle or any such recepticle, there we notice that peculiar

sound, and that we give the name amphoric or cavernous. . . .
What do you understand by vesicular breathing? What are its
characteristics?

When the student replied that it sounds like air going through a
small space, Dock elaborated: "What kind of a small space? It sounds
like a soft breeze through the trees. It must be free of all blowing." Then:

DOCK: Here is one important sign; listen anywhere around
there and tell me what you hear.

STUDENT: I could hear, on inspiration, something; it seems to
me to be a sort of thumping, a kind of rapping sound.

DOCK: That is not what I mean. Perhaps it sounds so common-
place that you would not think it worth mentioning. You hear the
heart sounds? Don't you think they are of an unusual distinctness?

STUDENT: Well, you would naturally hear them though.

DOCK: That is just the point. Do you naturally hear them there?
You don't hear them so well at a distance from the heart. Now
what physical changes in there would make you hear them? Well,
infiltration, consolidation, increased density, anything that will
increase the density of the lung will conduct the sound better.

Dock asked another student to listen to the spoken voice.

STUDENT: I think it is more distinct and not so clear.

DOCK: You didn't notice anything else? I don't like to force people to believe things like that, but it seems to me when you listen
along there, as you strike this line, a new quality comes into the
sound like a vibration, as if from a hollow instrument that was
cracked and as if it resembles bleating. That crackling quality
is what characterizes egophony. . . . What did you get her to
whisper?

STUDENT: One, two, three.

DOCK: There is much difference what syllables they whisper so
that it is not altogether a matter of taste although some people use
different syllables from those we use here, ninety-nine for exam-

ple. But in saying one, two, three the syllable "three" brings out the characteristics of the whispered voice better than almost any other syllable. Thirty-three brings it out too, and because of its explosive nature insures a hissing character in the three. Ninety-nine does not insure that.

X-Ray Diagnosis

The first mention of the use of X rays in the diagnosis of tuberculosis of the lungs occurred in 1902. Later when Dock showed the X ray of a patient the student had diagnosed as having "beginning tuberculosis," Dock said: "There is a slight cloudiness in the apex region; but ordinarily a skiagraph including the apices is not likely to be useful unless the disease is well advanced." Other attempts were frustrated by breakdown of the equipment, but the next year Dock could say:

It will be interesting to examine the skiagraph; although our facilities for examining them are not the best. This is a skiagraph of this patient and in as much as it is very easy to make a skiagraph look like almost anything I should say that this was a very good one. Taking this to be the right side, there is a shadow over the upper part showing increased density there, and also along the inner part. Here you see increased density all over. . . . In other words it is a skiagraph of a very extensive interstitial process.

Dock could read a skiagraph, but students had not been taught to do so.

DOCK: How about the skiagraph, Baxter? What does it show?

STUDENT: The left side of the thorax is much smaller than the other.

DOCK: And what else?

STUDENT: It looks clear.

DOCK: We always reverse the colors because of course that is the negative; the white is the shadow.

In 1907 Dock showed both AP and PA views of the chest of the law student who had been spitting blood a few months before. Dock saw pleurisy on one side and extensive infiltration of the lung on the other side. Dock had seen day-to-day changes. "So what he needs is not any particular climate, but treatment for his exact condition." The outcome in the next three or four weeks is very uncertain, and "it is likely that the outcome will be the wrong way." The list of graduates of the law school does not contain this student's name.

Laboratory Diagnosis of Tuberculosis: Sputum

Dock said early examination of sputum is important.

There is a very important fallacy about that examination that I would wish to urge you to avoid. Spitting or expectoration is not after all a normal condition. I am not talking about the secretion of the mouth or of the nose that gets down into the pharynx, but of the stuff that comes up through the larynx, and in such a way that there is every reason to see that it does come from the thorax and not from anywhere else. Anybody who does that is sick. In a large proportion of such cases they have a sickness that may be recognized by examination of the sputum, and so I say that when they have such a condition they should have the sputum examined; to be sure they should have a physical examination even before that. Very often for various reasons they don't do that. But in the case of sputum, the remarkable thing is that it isn't examined. For example, numerous specialists who devote themselves to lung disease in the west say that not more than 40 per cent. of patients ever had their sputum examined; yet most of them were sent out by doctors because they have a certain lung disease. . . . The first examination may be negative and a later one may be easily positive. And those of you who do microscopic work when you get out, and I hope all of you will, whenever you examine a specimen and don't find anything can only say it means nothing at all. . . . It is the easiest thing

UNIVERSITY HOSPITAL

DEPARTMENT OF INTERNAL MEDICINE

SPUTUM EXAMINATION

Name ....Date....................

In-patient, No.................Out-patient, No.................

Extra ....Dr. ....Diagnosis ....

Amount ....Sample ....24 Hours ....

Color ....Character ....Consistence...............

Odor ....Reaction ....

Cells: ......pavement epithelium.........alveolar cells...........

    dust cells ....heart-failure cells...............

    leukocytes, mononuclear ....

        "   polynuclear ....

        "   eosinophile ....

    colloid ....myelin bodies...................

    red blood cells ....

Tubercle bacilli: method used............Number...............

    appearance ....

....

Other bacteria, number and kind..............................

Elastic tissue, kind and quantity..............................

Spirals, kind and number ....

Charcot-Leyden crystals ....

Other findings ....

....

....

....

....

....

....

               Examined by...........................

FIGURE 14. Form used in Dock's department for reporting examination of the sputum.

in the world to get if the patient is raising anything. I always tell people the best thing to do is to get a wide mouthed bottle, say a quinine or morphine bottle, and then have the bottle with them when they first begin to get up and move around to carefully expectorate into the bottle, and to do that without having any tobacco in the mouth and before eating, and also to urge them to keep the mouth clean by using a tooth brush. . . . You tell them you just want what they cough up and they proceed to give you the remnants of their breakfast. We have to explain that we want not his breakfast or the pickings from his teeth or tobacco but just what he gets from his chest. There is no use talking of the thorax; some of them don't even know what the chest means, then you have to show them. All these things are important if we ever intend to push back the diagnosis and attain early and successful treatment of such a condition.

When tubercle bacilli were found in a sample of sputum, Dock said there are many possibilities of a mistake. "We have a patient with t.b.c. whose sputum is filled with bacilli, and it might be he got that patient's cup." Bacilli might be transferred in the laboratory by forceps, or the cover slip might not have been cleaned properly. Dock said the first thing to do if the sputum is negative is to be sure the carbolfuchsin is all right. "Whenever you have covers that you know are full of t.b.'s a good thing to do is to mark the slide or cover and put it in a box for control at some future time. Then when you have a case that is suspicious and the first slide is negative, take one of the old preparations, stain it up and look at it."

Tuberculosis was finally diagnosed in a patient after a long physical examination, and tubercle bacilli were found in the sputum only after repeated search. "It shows that you should not be satisfied with negative results, but continue the examination as long as sputum is to be had."

In his search for tubercle bacilli Dock often injected questionable pleuritic fluid into a rabbit or a guinea pig. Once he showed students how to biopsy an enlarged lymph gland in a young girl's neck. Part of the tissue was to be injected into a rabbit, and Dock said such a test should have been done three years before.

A student found "excessive cells" in the urine of a patient with Potts' disease, and he suggested they might be smegma bacilli. Dock questioned him.

> STUDENT: I have never seen smegma [bacilli].
>
> DOCK: It is high time you saw them. You ought to have looked at those cells; those were very important, because the whole subject of acid-fast bacilli in the urine is important. One man examined a woman's urine, found things that looked like tb's, and made a diagnosis of tuberculosis; he found pain in the kidney region, which is not hard to do, had the kidney extirpated, and found it was negative; and then it was found that there are all kinds of germs that stain like this, and that can be found on mucous membranes, in ascites, and in sputum. It is important to understand the simplest matters about this.

Then Dock told how to get urine from men and women without contamination, and he described the characteristics of smegma bacilli that had been worked out by his colleague Murray Cowie, distinguishing them from tubercle bacilli.[7]

Diagnosis of Tuberculosis: The Tuberculin Test

For early diagnosis of tuberculosis Dock relied more on the tuberculin test than on the diazo reaction. The diazo reaction often becomes positive only in advanced stages of the disease, and then "it is of grave prognostic importance; 60 per cent die within six months after the diazo reaction occurs in the urine." In Germany a patient with a positive diazo reaction is not admitted to a state sanatorium because there is better use for the space. Dock said:

> Tuberculin is used a great deal at the present time [1904] as a diagnostic agent. There are a great many kinds of tuberculin in the market. But the tuberculin that is understood when you don't mention any other name is what is known as the old Koch's tuberculin, tuberculinum Kochin. It comes in little bottles like this,

which hold one c.c. and sell for $1.50 or $1.25 each. It is brownish liquid, about the color of a weak Gram's solution and almost watery in consistency. It is used in very small quantities, a diagnostic dose is a mg. To give it use a pipette graduated in hundredths of a c.c.; then make the average dilution in weak carbolic water and use that for injection. Ordinarily you give it in the upper part of the back, and it ordinarily produces no sign where you give it; but within twelve to thirty hours or more after you give the test, you have the reaction. The test here was given at eight o'clock one evening, and at six o'clock the next evening had reached its height. The characteristic curve, going up markedly, shows that the reaction here was perfect. . . . Never give the tuberculin unless there is some disease in a person, the nature of which should be cleared up; and never give it to a person who has distinct TBc with TB's and elastic tissue [in the sputum]. It is unnecessary, and one should not do unnecessary things to sick people.

The test is positive if the temperature rises. "There is no use trying to give the test if there is a fever; it makes it impossible to interpret the curve. Try to get the temperature about normal."

Dock thought a reaction of tuberculous tissue to tubercilin causes the temperature to rise. Once in 1907 a student presented a patient with what he thought was beginning tuberculosis.

DOCK: How do you know?

STUDENT. There is consolidation; the left apex is one inch above the clavicle; she has broncho-vasicular breathing. Vesicular breathing below is harsh; she has increased spoken voice; slight rales in the left apex; dulness on both sides; lagging.

DOCK: That is a formidable list of signs.

The patient's sputum was negative, but Dock said that was unimportant. The patient's temperature had risen after 1 mg of tuberculin.

DOCK (to student): When you found she was going to have the test what you should have done was to see her the next morning and find out whether she had had symptoms; whether she was dizzy, sick nauseated, had pain in the bones and muscles as if she was going to have grip, and they don't need to be very severe. The point is whether she had them at all, and whether they came on at a new event. Then you should have examined her, and ausculted her very carefully with reference to the condition she had before, and then you should have come up between classes and examined her again, and you should have come back at one o'clock and then at four, every time carefully ausculting her and making notes of the things you discovered, because to find a curve like that the nurse has worked out on the chart is only a part of the diagnosis. The most important point is not the fever and not the malaise, but the minute changes that take place in the diseased focus that are of the most importance. So you missed a chance and nobody else who has had a similar opportunity should not neglect it.

Dullness appeared in another patient's lungs after a tuberculin test, and Dock said the tuberculin might have caused a local reaction. At autopsy chronic pulmonary tuberculosis and recent miliary tuberculosis of liver and spleen were discovered. These reactions may have been the reason physicians were wary of the test.

Dock remarked:

Just before he [a tuberculous patient] came in here he said that the doctor who sent him here told him that the medicine that we inject often made the disease worse. His doctor has an idea that has been widespread and still there is very little ground for it. The idea at first was that the injection would liberate the bacilli from the foci and give the patient miliary tuberculosis. According to that idea you would expect the disease to be commoner now than before tuberculin was discovered. As a matter of fact that is not the case.

Nevertheless, Dock said of one patient: "She may have a latent case of tuberculosis in the course of encapsulation and injection of tuberculin may aggravate rather than benefit the condition."

In 1902 when a temperature rise was still the criterion of a positive tuberculin test, James Arneill said that it would be wise to give the test to a great many "normal patients" in the hospital. There is no evidence that was done, but by 1907 when it had become a skin test, Dock said that Dr. Smithies will give the "calmet" [Calmette] tuberculin test to the whole class. Also, "I understand you all want that and you certainly ought to be gratified in so harmonious a wish and, I may say, so admirable a wish."

In 1906 Dock used Wright's opsonin index,[8] but he apparently was having trouble.

> Of course such a case is a useful one for the opsonin test, but it is not easy to be working with the tuberculin opsonin index, and tuberculin carefully used gives a good deal more than the opsonin men seem to admit. . . . because by following the temperature and local reaction we have some guides that have proved pretty satisfactory, quite as satisfactory it might be said so far as the opsonin index itself.

Tuberculosis at Other Sites

In 1895 through 1908 Michigan deaths from tuberculosis were for disease in the

Thoracic cavity	20,858
Abdomen	1,957
Joints	122
Spine	82
Cranial cavity	61.[9]

Consequently, most of the tuberculous patients seen on Dock's service had tuberculosis of the lungs, sometimes with extension into the larynx. A few had tuberculous peritonitis. Dock demonstrated only one or two patients with tuberculosis of the kidneys or testicles, for those patients were handled by the surgeons. Surgeons also dealt with disease of the joints, and such patients appeared on Dock's wards only when they were referred with a question of extension of the disease to the lungs or in one instance to the meninges.

Dock had firm opinions on the treatment of tuberculous peritonitis:

A great many people say it is a medical disease. Tuberculosis of the peritoneum is not so very uncommon. They have very instructive histories, somewhat vague although highly suggestive, and at other times very distinct and very misleading; sometimes they have been brought in with appendicitis, and what they had was peritonitis without any diseased appendix. You see an abdomen that looks somewhat bloated. Now all those cases require very careful examination and they are comparatively easy to examine if you suspect the possible cause of the trouble. But if you think merely dyspepsia and don't look at the abdomen, you are likely to overlook some very important diagnostic signs. If you examine such patients, you find beside distention you can nearly always detect free fluid, but the distention is very often difficult. It is bound down so that it is not free and sometimes changes rapidly. Of course, in some cases you can feel lumps, masses corresponding to a thickened omentum or in some cases corresponding to adhesions. . . . It is a clinical fact that many patients get well of tuberculous peritonitis without any treatment. That is a fact nobody can deny, but anybody who would depend on a possibility of that kind ought logically to allow every disease to go untreated and such a person has no business in the profession of medicine. I dare say you are all posted [by Dr. Nancrede] in the history of operative treatment of tuberculous peritonitis, so that I may be going over familiar ground.

Dock did go over familiar ground, and then he said:

In regard to the details, there is a difference of opinion. There are people who believe the way to do is to open the abdomen, letting out everything there, and wash out with large quantities of normal saline solution. Others think all that is necessary is to let the fluid out. . . . How the operation does good we cannot answer, but that it is good has been demonstrated too often to doubt. For example one person had masses as big as your hand, and we had very little hope she could get over the operation. But she not only got over the operation well and although she had pulmonary symptoms at the time of the operation, she got over those too; and now, after nine years is alive and has been working all the time.

On April 10, 1901, Dock was out of town, and James Arneill took the clinic. Arneill said: "The opinion of the profession is somewhat divided upon the advisability of operation for tubercular peritonitis." In the margin Dock wrote in pencil:

No!

G.D.

Tuberculin Therapy

On October 7, 1904, Dock demonstrated a young Negro girl from Gary, Indiana, who had first been seen in the neurology clinic and then in the gynecological clinic. He said: "She was operated upon for something else, but Dr. Peterson, with his usual Sherlock Holmes sense, got after the appendix and after that was taken out found it had tuberculosis." Dock described the girl's family history: her mother had a running discharge from the axilla, and two sisters coughed a great deal. One of the sisters had enlarged glands in the neck. A tuberculin test was followed by chills, sweating, and severe pains all over the body. The temperature rose to 101.6°F and remained high for an unusually long time. Dock thought the prognosis was poor, but when he demonstrated her again on December 2, 1904, she was about to be discharged home. She had been treated with ascending doses of tuberculin, up to 1,600 mg, and she had had no reaction above 100°. Said Dock: "We expect to get up to the point where they do not react to enormous doses, and then it is considered good practice to stop." The girl should now have ordinary hygienic treatment and return in two months to be examined again.

In 1907 Dock had stopped using such large doses of tuberculin. He told the class:

> The history of the use of tuberculin is a very interesting one. Probably all of you are too young to remember when the tubercle bacillus was discovered. Everybody thought somebody would discover the antidote and everybody would immediately get well. It took ten years to find the promised antidote and when that was published the excitement was tremendous. People all over the world

sold their things and traveled half the circumference of the earth to get to Berlin. . . . It was considered as good as radium water today. Anybody who had a bottle of tuberculin had all sorts of unfortunate wretches following him; just as now for 5000 miles about Ann Arbor anyone who has a pain in the mammary gland wants to have radium water. . . . Accidents which followed from tuberculin were such that it drove people from using it. Nobody knew how to use it. They thought if a little was good, a lot was better so they gave patients all they could afford. It had very severe reactions; it was very expensive; the patient had fever and vomiting and great prostration. But a lot of men had favorable experiences and kept on using tuberculin. Nearly everybody else got so frightened that they stopped altogether—I was among that class myself.

Then Dock described the revival of the use of tuberclin after "Dr. Goetsch in Germany" published results he had obtained when he had used small doses of tuberculin in early cases of tuberculosis.[10] Dock said:

The improvement in using it was in using it not so much as to cause a severe reaction,—1/10 of a mg. would keep them from getting a severe reaction, and then the dose was doubled unless the indications were severe. If there was just a slight rise, instead of increasing the dose the next injection was the same as before. That is the way it was used in the last six years and is used here, with encouraging results in the cases we treated. . . . Just at present this treatment is undergoing another modification and that is in the direction of still smaller doses. This is due to opsonin therapy. The people who use it have an idea that brave men never lived before Agamemnon. . . . There is another point in regard to small doses. It is interesting especially because so far-sighted a man as [Richard] Cabot has fallen into error. He takes the ground that giving small doses of tuberculin is exactly the same as giving a homeopathic dose of medicine.

Dock said homeopaths must have laughed in their sleeves or even more visibly when they heard Cabot say that. Also, Dock said:

Another point shows how a man may be in error, even one from Back Bay who passes the house Oliver Wendell Holmes lived in, although if he ever read Dr. Holmes "taking a club to Kill [blank]"[11] it is hard to see how he would. But it grieves me to see such a man who is not only Demonstrator in Medicine at Harvard but has the Chair of Philosophy there, leave his premise and make such a statement.

On December 12, 1899, Dock prescribed cod liver oil and creosote, 10 to 15 drops t.i.d., for a girl of fifteen whose prognosis was "serious but not unfavorable." He did not continue the 5% solution of nucleinic acid her physician had been giving her.

Nucleinic acid, nor nuclein, was an alkaline alcoholic extract of yeast, and since 1893 it had been Dean Victor Vaughan's favorite remedy for almost every infectious disease. Vaughan himself did not make white cell counts, but he thought nuclein acted by stimulating leucocytosis. When he reported results of nuclein therapy for twenty-four tuberculous patients, Vaughan wrote with his own emphasis:

> Even when tuberculosis is of long standing, and when the extent of tissue involved is great, *so long as secondary infection with pyogenic germs has not occurred*, the proper use of the remedy may *retard* (I do not say arrest) the progress of the disease. . . . Already some physicians are supplying tuberculous patients with hypodermic syringes and solutions of nucleinic acid, and telling them to go ahead and treat themselves.[12]

Fifteen months later a student asked:

> How about nuclein?
>
> DOCK: For a couple of years we used it to a great extent. I was never able to demonstrate a marked leucocytosis from the effect of nuclein. It is active but certainly not a specific. I think it is something of a fad.

Telling the Patient

Dock said that the patient deserves much more careful treatment now than when consumption was thought to be incurable and that the patient must be told in the beginning that his disease requires long and careful treatment; otherwise he will think you are not doing all that is necessary.

> Everybody old enough should be carefully informed as to what kind of a disease he has and what the probable course of this disease is likely to be. It is not long since patients with consumption were carefully kept in ignorance of what they had with the idea that they would be frightened. A bad prognosis should never be made until the patient is on his last legs. I had a striking example of the importance of that when I first went into a hospital, and where I was anxious to learn from more experienced people as much as possible about prognosis of disease. I asked an old nurse about the prognosis of a patient with consumption; how long she thought he would live. The nurse told me she never gave them up until they got cold. . . . So that I would say in such a case the prognosis ought to be an unfavorable one; but, at the same time, I would not in practice make an unfavorable one to the patient, because where possibility of improvement is admitted, it is very much to the patient's advantage to take a favorable view of the prognosis. If you tell him he can't get over it, he probably will not and, on the other hand, if you cheer him up he will get better, but the relatives ought to know there is serious danger.

Home Treatment

Most tuberculous patients in Michigan were treated at home, and "all over the state we have not only a hundred little houses but a thousand little houses that have one consumptive in them." Dock asked what is to be done if a patient has tuberculosis "in a form fairly well established and not very actively developing and is in a condition offering a very good chance of recovery." He answered himself by saying:

> One of the great problems in such a case is, what the patient can do. He is married and has a family, that is two children, and he would find it difficult to leave home under any conditions, proba-

bly impossible to leave with his family. . . . [T]hey don't have to go away from home to get well. The reason that they do better is that they do more things away from home; they subject themselves to discipline, that is, they live the way they ought to,—eat the way they ought to, sleep the way they ought, exercise and rest they way they ought to. But if a patient is willing to spend the same kind of life at home, then there is no reason why he should not get along as well in Podunk as in Arizona for instance.

"Milk, eggs, meat, and fresh vegetables after all form the most useful diet," and "you give them the food you would give to people you are try-ing to fatten, a diet highly nutritious and easily absorbed." The patient should be weighed every week under the same conditions and on the same scale. "He must get all the fresh air he can. Whether God's pure air or your or my pure air doesn't make any difference as far as the applica-tion is concerned. The point is that pure air anywhere can do a great deal of good. . . . Of course we use that treatment not to kill germs but for the wide spread stimulating effect on the individual." To get fresh air, the patient should be out-of-doors during the bright part of the day.

But I would not have him out-of-doors on his back because he would have a cold back or get hypostatic congestion or his feet get so cold that he would have to be unnecessarily covered up with clothes. But in a reclining chair he could stay out all day long, with a hot water bag to his feet and a blanket or blankets around his legs and hot drinks, milk or any other hot drink every couple of hours. . . . A patient out of doors must have everything done under the covers, the urinal and bed pan placed under them, properly warmed of course.

If the patient sleeps on a screened porch, use a wide bed, and keep the covers tucked in. Put paper under the mattress so that the mattress is not cold, and put papers between layers of covers so that the patient can remain warm without uncomfortable weight on him.

The amount of exercise that [a] patient can stand must be care-fully discovered by practice and then [the] patient should be en-couraged to take that. Harm has been done by overworking tuberculous people, although many have recovered in spite of their overwork. It is good for well people to become tired but no sick people are made well by getting tired.

In Germany, patients walk through the woods singing, "but we don't burst into melody as they do."

Dock scorned the doctor who "was brought up to think that the patient must have cod liver oil, or if he has a fever, an antipyretic; if night sweats, large quantities of medicine; if a cough, at least half a dozen different medicines in one bottle." Cough syrups should never be used unless the patient is about to die, and then they will do no harm by ruining his digestion further. "Very often giving a patient a glass of milk or water at bed time will keep away night sweats. Very often a basin of water put under the bed will keep away night sweats. This is still used in some parts of the country."

Dock knew the problems of home treatment, and when discussing one patient he said:

> She needs the care of almost the whole time of another person. Also if she lives as the average individual she has four or five other people living with her or four or five children clambering over the bed, sometimes the whole family even are obliged to live in one room. But even where there is plenty of room it is not uncommon to find all the children, ranging in age from one to eighteen, lounging about on the bed clothes where there is dried sputum, and, if the patient coughs, danger of drop infection. So that altogether the problem is a serious one and it is usually hopeless in the case of poor patients.

Going West

Before 1907 the alternative to home treatment was to go West, and Dock wondered whether to send a woman to Texas, where "you can see farther and see less than in any other country."

Dock said never to send a patient away from home unless you know he will do better away. In a majority of cases, whether a person can go to a better climate is a financial rather than a medical question, and unless the patient can stay a number of months the benefits are not likely to be permanent. Dock said:

> In regard to the place, a great deal of error exists in the minds of people at large. For example, thirty or forty years ago, if people had lung disease, they were sent to Italy or Florida because at that time it was supposed that a warm climate was the climate for consumptives. Later it became the custom to send patients to places with high altitudes, and the people went to Switzerland, Colorado or New Mexico.

Another idea was that there should be only a slight difference in temperature between night and day.

> For a person who needs stimulation it is better to get them into higher altitude about 3000 ft. If he has no fibroid tendency, then he may be sent as high as a mile and in many cases much higher. If he has a weak heart or extensive lung disease, to send him to such an altitude as that—although it might affect him well in some ways, will have bad effects in other ways. So try to find out the place that will be proper for your patient to live and you have to spend time investigating climatic conditions in different parts of the country, and they are not always easy to procure.

Once Dock had a physician from California describe the varieties of climate there. Dock said that classes scatter, and medical classmates should keep in touch with each other to exchange such information.

> Then when you find that a patient has to go away always be sure that where he is going he will not be worse off, even with a better climate, than he will be at home. A place with merely a good climate will not do. Patients are sent by the thousands to various western points and have no idea whether they are going to the right place. They may get in a place that is too high, too dry, too dusty, where there are no comforts at all, and the first thing they know they have a local disease as the result of bad food or bad water.

The patients needs continued medical attention. After you select the part of the country, Dock said: "then send him to the care of some physician living in that part of the country, to whom the patient may go to be examined and have the details of future life laid out for him." In exceptional instances, "[i]f he is strong and hasn't too much local disease in the lungs, then he can take some risks. He can go to a ranch or anything that will take him thousands of miles from medical care; but many can't stand that sort of neglect." All patients do better if they have something to do. Dock remarked:

> One of the easiest things is to work on a goat ranch or a chicken ranch. A goat ranch is the easiest. A sheep ranch requires a great deal of activity, especially in bad weather. [A] patient on a goat ranch has enough to do to keep him from thinking of his own discomfort. People with mechanical trades can often work at ordinary trades in such places.

At another time Dock said:

> They may run a ranch, or garden, or drive a stage coach. For example, I have now a high school teacher—one of the best in the state—who is driving a mail coach in South Arizona. Although [the] patient sometimes gets a pain in the lung when the horses pull, he is able to keep at work with great benefit. But it must be remembered that in the new parts of the country stage driving is a healthy and lucrative occupation, and I expect to see him judge of the supreme court in the state to which he has gone as a stage driver.

Being away has its problems: "It is a well known fact that many persons have been sent away and been so homesick and fed on such poor food that they die long before they might have at home, with good care."

Tuberculous patients do not need medicines, Dock said, but because they think medicines are necessary they spend money foolishly on "cures." Dock thought one man had been taking patent medicines. He had spent the winter in Salt Lake City, and Dock questioned him about conditions in Zion.

DOCK. Didn't you meet other people like yourself?

PATIENT: Oh, eight out of ten people cough there. They always laughed there and spoke of it as a cigarette cough. Everybody smokes cigarettes; I saw men sixty years old smoking them.

DOCK: Didn't any barker stop you in the street and offer to treat you? Usually a man out there is stopped by a runner for a doctor.

PATIENT: Usually I saw nothing out there but saloons, gambling houses and boarding houses.

Sanatorium Care

Dock wanted a special isolation ward for tuberculous patients built as part of the University Hospital, and he thought such a ward should be part of every community hospital.[13] Patients could receive special care, and because they were isolated they would not endanger other patients. Only patients with incipient tuberculosis would be admitted; patients in later stages would be excluded. An effort to persuade the legislature to provide the ward failed in 1902; instead, a state sanatorium was opened at Howell, Michigan, a few miles north of Ann Arbor, in 1907.[14]

In 1905 Dock told the students:

As you all know agitation is going on for the building of some sort of institution for the care of consumptives. In Germany the development of these institutions has been rapid for a number of reasons. First, because they were suggested early; second the accident insurance laws, and insurance of working people make[s] it possible to spend large sums of money in this way. . . . In Germany, for example, they have found it cheaper to put men in a sanatorium to treat them than to let them go. . . . In this country many institutions have been built and no doubt many more will be built. Most of them are institutions that can only be used by those with an amount of money. In the Adirondacks there is such an institution where the patient has to pay $5.00 per week. If the patient is poor, it has to be paid just the same.

As an aside, Dock said:

I perhaps should say that the difference between sanitarium and sanatorium is partly a verbal one. It is a rule in English to derive words from the Latin, say, by using the adjective whereas the Germans have the fashion of using the noun.

Several times while the Howell hospital was being planned and built, Dock talked to the students about how patients are treated in a tuberculosis sanatorium. On January 10, 1905, he discovered that Dr. Elliott of the Ontario tuberculosis sanatorium was in town.[15] Dock said that "if it had not been for my gentle and retiring disposition I would have him talk all the time this afternoon" about a great many interesting and instructive things, including tropical diseases. "[B]ut for the majority some of the work he is doing now at Gravenhurst in the Muskoka region in the treatment of tuberculosis will be more valuable."

Elliott told the students that one in eight persons in Canada and the United States dies of tuberculosis. But "we must look upon tuberculosis as one of the most curable of chronic diseases," and he described the Muskoka regimen in detail. Seventy-five per cent of patients who enter in the incipient stage recover. Elliott said: "Some recover at the end of several months; others at from one to two years; and still others have been struggling hard to get well for seven or eight years, and are getting just about well at the end of this time. Large proportions of cases will have cavity formation; practically none of them recover." Elliott ended by saying: "As pulmonary tuberculosis is a disease from which medical students and physicians are prone to suffer, it is incumbent upon students to place themselves as far as possible in proper hygienic conditions, and where infection is incurred we must keep our bodily health up to the highest point possible so that if we have the disease it may not be dangerous."

The Antituberculosis Movement

In 1906 Dock told the students:

Just at this, time and in fact in the last two or three years, there is great activity all over the country in the formation of associations for the purpose of combating tuberculosis; that is one of their favorite words, "combating", and nearly all of these associations have the purpose of combating the disease on a large scale, i.e., of collecting together large quantities of patients and putting them on the treatment that everybody believes now is the best treatment. But there are certain fallacies connected with this movement that it is highly important for young doctors to consider. The movement at the present time does not consider enough the need of education in the detection of these cases. Why are they recognized so late? Chiefly because they don't look for them early. The problem is still more of an individual problem for the practicing physician than it is for the association. If they looked for tuberculosis of the lungs as they look for ovarian tumors or other kinds of surgical or gynecological tumors it would be better. It is said that the science of operative medicine is in advance of internal medicine. It must be admitted that we are not so keen to search for internal disease as they are for a fibroid of the uterus, for example. But that is the fault simply of the practice, and I strongly suspect that the association movement will tend to relieve us of the responsibilities that we ought to feel, and we will say "the General National Association will handle this thing for us; we don't need to handle it at all."

Just before he left Michigan in 1908 Dock told the students:

The public takes up all sorts of hygienic fads as all other ephemeral things, and very often they get over them almost as soon as they take them up, which is an excellent thing when the fad is not a good one. It is important when the fad of short skirts and low heels give place to the fad of long skirts and high heels; but it would be very important if this other fad that has been taken up by all classes of people is allowed to go the way of the corset of yesterday. Societies are being formed everywhere, and if not guided by the doctor will become useless or even pernicious, but if guided by doctors who know what they are doing then the gain to the community will be very great. And this gain to the community represents gain to the doctor. There is a lot of silly trash being uttered that the movement is going to take the bread out of the mouth of the doctor. But by taking up so important a piece of work and by showing good sense, perseverance, enthusiasm and knowledge of the subject, by doing that the young doctor has a way of making himself favorably known such as he might not be able to accomplish in any other way in years.

SMALLPOX

13.

JAMES ARNEILL SAID THE
University Hospital was overwhelmed with smallpox in 1900–1901.[1] If
the reports are correct, it was even worse in Michigan in the next year.[2]

YEAR	REPORTED CASES	REPORTED DEATHS	DEATHS PER 100,000
1898	32	1	0.04
1899	139	6	0.3
1900	694	9	0.4
1901	5,088	31	1.3
1902	7,086	40	1.6
1904	5,753	24	0.9
1905	2,985	74	2.9
1906	1,240	3	0.1
1907	1,712	8	0.3
1908	2,306	8	0.3

Dock said:

For smallpox have been very common ever since the glorious war
with Spain; in fact, that was one of the causes of increasing smallpox here. . . . Just why there should be so much smallpox here is an
interesting thing, one that should be a matter of the most serious
reproach to any state, but it is only one of a number of things that
indicates to a philosophical mind the very thin veneering of our
so-called civilization. It is just as bad to have smallpox as to have
leprosy or to have, for example, the itch. We all look down with

237

contempt on the poor Viennese because they all have the itch, but it is no worse for them to have the itch than for us to have the smallpox.

At another time Dock wrote:

A country that sees its citizens killed off in their best years by typhoid fever without making a move to prevent the disease is not likely to pay much attention to the loss of a few hundred people a year from smallpox.[3]

A Diagnostic Error

A patient was admitted on Wednesday, December 12, 1900, and demonstrated by Dock the next Friday afternoon. The patient had a bright, flushed appearance and a continuous high fever. Dock pressed down with a cover glass on the sharply circumscribed spots on the patient's abdomen to show that they returned when the cover glass was removed. They "are highly characteristic, perfectly characteristic of typhoid spots. You may go a long time before you see any as pretty as this. You can make the diagnosis [of typhoid fever] without any misgivings."

By Saturday night misgivings had accumulated. The patient now had a papular eruption on the back of the neck, the cheeks, and the forehead. The patient's temperature was not affected by bathing, but it fell suddenly from 104–105°F to normal. There was no diazo reaction, and the Widal test was positive only at 1:20 dilution. On Tuesday Dock explained the early mistake. It was unusual for a smallpox eruption to appear on the abdomen first. The patient had an enlarged spleen, and that too is unusual in smallpox. The pulse instead of being above 100 was below 90 and was not dicrotic. Dock had not known that the patient had traveled in a country where there had been smallpox the year before, but "If he had come from Custer, Ludington, or the Upper Peninsula, one might think that he had smallpox."

Now it is important to take precautions and to prevent alarm. The number of attendants had been diminished, and the patient had been moved to the isolation ward on Sunday.

The official history of the university described the ward:

At the time the Catherine Street Hospitals were erected in 1891, a small shack on the property . . . was taken over and used as a laundry. With the removal of the heating plant to a new building in 1897, the laundry was moved into a new building, and at a cost of $200 the old building was fitted up as a separate contagious disease hospital and equipped with furniture for an additional sum of $36.15.[4]

Dock objected very strongly to calling it "the pest house"; he preferred "North Ward." Dock urged his students to observe patients with contagious diseases through the glass windows, and on occasion he took the students with him after class to see a smallpox patient. There was no danger, but "there is this about it, if you see these patients and then go with some other person who develops smallpox in a couple of weeks, then you are likely to be accused of having spread smallpox."

Dock himself had trouble diagnosing smallpox when the disease was mild and when "you can call them varioloid if you wish." In 1902 a woman with smallpox was sent to the University Hospital with her physician's diagnosis of chicken pox, despite the fact that there were ten cases of smallpox in her village. In discussing the difficulty of distinguishing between smallpox and chicken pox in their early stages, Dock said:

It is important for every student to see such cases and see them as often as possible. We are not strict about those things around the middle west as in some other places. In Philadelphia doctors have been fined for not recognizing [smallpox]; a classmate of mine was fined $200 because he was not able to make the diagnosis, and some of you may get into a town where they have those same rigid ideas.

Nevertheless,

when I make a differentiation between chicken pox and smallpox I have to admit that, personally, I am far from convinced that chicken pox and smallpox are entirely distinct diseases. Kaposi believed to the last that chicken pox is only a mild form of smallpox; and it is an interesting fact that people who don't believe so rarely have the experience he had. Having seen 5000 cases, he admitted there were some things he did not know; yet some who have seen 50 cases think they know it all, which is a dangerous thing to do.

Dock recommended Kaposi's book to the students.[5]

Treatment

Dock observed:

> A word in regard to the treatment. It is purely nursing. The best thing that a smallpox patient can have is an intelligent, cool-handed, kind-hearted nurse. I think we are fortunate in having for this man a man whose race is noted for its kindness of heart and a race that furnishes a very large number of very good nurses. He has come through smallpox and had it himself so that he knows a little about it, and no doubt that with the supervision that we can give him he ought to take good care of him.

A patient with smallpox was bathed every four or five hours with a 1:500 solution of bichloride of mercury. Bathing reduced tension in the skin, and the mercury solution reduced chances of secondary infection. The vesicles might dry up without becoming pustules. Dock thought there was little chance that enough mercury would be absorbed to cause constitutional symptoms, but in one instance a smallpox patient had what looked like mercury erythema. A patient was fed a liquid diet, and he used a potassium chlorate mouthwash. If he had trouble sleeping, Dock, who said he was not in favor of shotgun therapy, gave him "20 grains of chloral, 40 of bromide and 20 of hyoscyamus each night" for two nights. When the patient was convalescent, he was frequently bathed with soft soap until the last evidence of desquamation had disappeared. If he recovered rapidly, he might be allowed "to get out inside the traditional six weeks that such a patient ought to be isolated."

Scarring

As an amateur medical historian, Dock knew the tradition that wrapping a smallpox patient in red cloth prevents scarring, and he owned a copy of John of Gaddesden's *Rosa Anglica* in which that fourteenth-century physician asserted that he had cured without scarring the son of an English king by wrapping the patient in red and hanging red cloth about the bed.[6] In Dock's time at Michigan, red-light treatment was being promoted by Niels Finsen, the Danish heliotherapist, who had written:

> In July, 1893, I proposed a new treatment for smallpox, which consists in placing the patients in rooms from which the chemical rays of the spectrum are excluded by interposing red glass or thick red cloth. The results of this method of treatment are that the vesicles as a rule do not enter upon the stage of suppuration, and that the patients get well with no scars at all, or at the most with extremely slight scarring.[7]

Others were skeptical, and so was Dock; he told his students he did not use the red-light treatment.

On February 1, 1901 the university student who had been misdiagnosed in December returned to the clinic so that the class could see him.

> DOCK: Although the present appearance of the patient is not what most people would want to have, I think on the whole he may be considered lucky. . . . You are going to lectures are you?
>
> PATIENT: Yes, sir.
>
> DOCK: They are not clearing out from you are they?
>
> PATIENT: Not very much.
>
> DOCK: I have seen street cars emptied by people in that condition getting aboard.

There had not been another case of smallpox in Ann Arbor because everyone had been careful. Dock said: "I am told that last year a patient in Detroit was taken in Harper Hospital and 30 students in the clinic contracted the disease and one of the students died. . . . I am strongly of the opinion that washing the hands after handling patients of all kinds is one of the safest ways of avoiding infection."

Dealing with an Epidemic

In 1904 there was another statewide epidemic, and smallpox prevailed in fifty Michigan communities. Dock said:

> There is a certain amount of alarm in town and that alarm can be quieted by an explanation by the student or doctor who comes into contact with such people. It will be the duty of every student to lay down the law in regard to vaccination. Only a few years ago a smallpox house was fired here while the smallpox patient was still in it. It behooves every senior medical student to consider how he should act and what he should do in such an emergency. You are looked on as fountains of wisdom, and are liable at boarding house tables and in Bible classes[8] to be asked about smallpox and vaccination and, if you have a ready answer, you will gain much credit. If all of you will resolve yourselves into a committee of one, it will probably have a good effect on the community, and the non–medical student body as it is called.

There were many cases of smallpox in Milan, Michigan, a town some twenty miles south of Ann Arbor, and a patient was brought from Milan to the University Hospital for an emergency appendectomy. She had been in a "horrible state of uncleanliness," swarming with lice and with an enormous number of nits in her hair. The nurse who washed her discovered she was a smallpox convalescent. Dock discussed the legal problems of transporting a smallpox patient from a country farmhouse to the hospital, and he said there was a moral duty to warn the hospital. She should have been coated with a "pretty strong bichloride solution" and wrapped in clean clothes and in sheets and blankets that had been baked in an oven at the risk of being scorched. She should have then been carried on a shutter. Two months later Dock demonstrated her scars and said she still had nits that threatened everyone in the vicinity. "Just how much and how persistent an effort has been made to eradicate them I cannot say because I haven't recently talked to the nurses about them. It requires persistence that one can hardly see outside a monkey cage."

At that time there were two men with smallpox in the isolation ward. They said they did not know where they got the disease. Dock said that may or may not be true. "They may decline to admit it because they wish to protect other people. They may have someone in their own homes who has a similar disease and they know it." One of the patients had been vaccinated three times, and a doctor had told him he was immune. Dock said: "If a doctor tells a patient that he is immune after a single trial or ten or twenty or thirty trials, he is telling something that is absolutely untrue in a scientific way, and rather close to criminal immorality in other ways."

Two weeks later there were more patients in the isolation ward. One was the wife of a man who had been admitted earlier, and another was a woman who had been taking her meals with seventy-five others in a large boarding house. Two engineering students had been eating at the same table while they had early smallpox eruptions. Dock remarked:

Of course we don't know how much closer contact there may have been. Eating utensils in the boarding house may have been infected and not properly cleaned. One would do well to observe at such times the German custom of jamming the fork through the napkin several times and rubbing the knife very vigorously on the table cloth.

And a week later:

Now we have a couple of very interesting phenomena brought to our attention lately; for example, a medical student is now in the other smallpox hospital, and this points a moral and teaches something. This man was seeing a patient who was sick, but not a medical student. The other student thought he was sick enough to see a doctor, and the doctor considered the possibility of smallpox but took the other diagnosis. This other individual, after being told by a doctor that he did not have smallpox, developed smallpox. I mention it not by way of criticism of the man who made the diagnosis, but I mention them because they point a moral, because they show how much better it would be in all cases, if possible, to carry out prophylactic treatment. The medical student had been vaccinated, and had been vaccinated at a time that should have made him immune to smallpox. Then, inasmuch as he had been exposed, he was vaccinated again. Both took. The second one was made just before the smallpox symptoms began. Of course that was too late to do anything except, perhaps, to diminish the severity of the infection.

Vaccination

In each of the smallpox epidemic years, or when a smallpox patient appeared at the University Hospital, there was what Dock called a "vaccination debauch." All doctors and nurses and their families and all medical students were vaccinated. If a medical student ate in a boarding house, an attempt was made to vaccinate all in the house as well. Dock said:

Everyone in Ann Arbor ought to be vaccinated. Smallpox is a disease that grows worse the more material it has to feed on. A large number of unprotected people in a town increases the danger. . . . In countries where people think about such things and where governments take as much pains to protect the human individual as they do their cattle, which rarely happens in a republic, people are not led to run the risk of an incomplete vaccination. . . . So try to suppress all those panicky ideas by showing you have confidence in your ability to protect yourself by vaccination or by showing the superiority that every doctor should have against such accidents as disease or death.

Nevertheless, Dock wrote:

What we need, in my opinion, is not compulsion, our first antidote against all evils, from corsets to obnoxious corporations, but an organized and scientific procedure that shall have the confidence of a large majority of the people.[9]

When he described the technique of vaccination, Dock said:

We notice that vaccination is frequently done in the most trivial and careless way. I have known doctors and physicians to vaccinate hundreds of people a day at 25 per, as they say; they tell the patient to put up his sleeve, make a scratch and place some of the vaccine in and let the patient go away. I think this is an immoral practice. . . . When you vaccinate have your hands clean, have the patient's arm clean and have a sterilized knife. Don't put any antiseptic on the arm for the more you rub it the greater is the likelihood of complications and the less likelihood there is of having a good take and instead of preventing abscess and gangrene, to bring it on.

Make two longitudinal incisions about one inch apart and three-quarters to one inch long with a sterile scalpel, not deep enough to draw blood in large drops. If the incision is too deep, make another. If the patient has been exposed to smallpox, make three or four incisions. Gently rub the vaccine in; do not grind it; and allow it to dry. Don't put on a dressing unless the patient is likely to contaminate it. Then use only a light protective dressing of sterile gauze. Shields are available in Germany but not yet in this country. Follow up by inspecting the site about eight days later. Encourage revaccination, and keep records![10] "Then we should take a proper view of the seriousness of the operation by making a legitimate charge for the services. To vaccinate for 25 cts., 50 cts., or a dollar is one of the most curious things that somebody can do. People who charge several dollars for opening an abscess will sit down and vaccinate for a quarter. So I always charge. I don't always get it, of course."

Dock described a successful take, and students had plenty of opportunity to see one. After a vaccination debauch, Dock inspected the arm of each member of the class, commenting freely:

There is a little too much irritation; it may have been rubbed too much or simply be an accident. . . . Here is something that is rather different from the others. This looks as if it was going to take but probably not very freely; you see the beginning of vesicles there, four in one scratch and others not so distinct. . . . That was cut too deep and too close together. . . . Well, those haven't begun yet, although it looks as if they might take a little. . . . Here is the method I object to. The trouble is here you have a thin scab over the place where the stuff was inserted; now if it takes around there, you can't have a typical sore. Moreover such a scab favors secondary infection.

And so on.

A student asked, "how young you should vaccinate children." Dock replied: "You can vaccinate them as soon as they are born, but a young child usually doesn't stand as much risk of smallpox as an older one but if, for example, I had to go and see children under six months [while treating smallpox patients], I would have them all vaccinated."

Failure to Protect and Complications

Patients with smallpox said they had been vaccinated. Dock stated:

I never tell people, for example, that vaccination is a sure protection against smallpox because we know it isn't, neither is smallpox, but that it is, on the whole, the best protection that we have. . . . People will say I have been vaccinated every year for so many years and it has never taken. In such cases, first, the vaccination may never have been effective. That is the usual explanation. There are cases, however, in which vaccination does not take place and people think they are immune, but nothing is more serious as an error than to say that such a person will not take smallpox again, because cases have been observed. For example, Dr. Osler failed to take vaccination but nevertheless took smallpox.

Glycerinated lymph had been on the market since 1891, and Dock preferred to use it rather than "points" or threads that had been soaked in lymph and dried.[11] Glycerination increases the quantity of vaccine available, and it kills some bacteria, the erysipelas streptococcus, for example. In the United States the supply of vaccine is unregulated, and vaccine is widely advertised without proof of efficacy. The Chicago Board of Health found that only 25% of preparations took. In one Ann Arbor epidemic, ten thousand parcels of vaccine had been used. One batch was good, but another was not. Makers should test their product, but they do not know the characteristic lesion. A government station for making and testing vaccine is highly desirable, or at least there should be government inspection.

Bacterial purity can be tested, but often it is not. Dock noted:

Three years ago there were nearly 100 cases of tetanus in this country from vaccination. It is all very well to say that in some of these cases the patients got tetanus germs themselves from their finger nails or clothes, yet we can't deny the fact that many of them came from the vaccine material because they were found in vaccine material from other sources. One man examined vaccine material from his own vaccine institution and out of 400, five gave tetanus cultures.

A patient whose vaccination had become infected was shown in the clinic, and after had had been removed Dock said he had been infected by dirty garments. "If such a patient came to you in private practice, you should tell him he must have clean clothes; but here where we vaccinate the patients whether they want to or not we can't do that." At another time a sentence in the transcript began: "C . . . . was extremely dirty . . ." Above this entry is written in Dock's hand: "The pat who died of tetanus," so the entry should read:

The patient who died of tetanus was extremely dirty, and probably in such a case there is always danger that the tetanus germs are there and will be scratched in by the patient; or if he hadn't died from infection of the smallpox, he probably would have scratched his foot on an old nail and died in that way. Not all cases of tetanus have been so clear in that respect.

MORE INFECTIOUS DISEASES

14.

DOCK DEMONSTRATED

very few cases of measles to his students, for most children with measles were cared for at home. In 1904 when there were 10,386 reported cases of measles in Michigan with a death rate of 7.0 per 100,000,[1] a child with an indistinct eruption on his face was brought to the University Hospital by his mother. Dock began his examination: "Now let us see his mouth. Over here we see little white spots not much bigger than the point of a pin with little red spots around them. You ought all to look at that. Take your fingers, turn the cheeks inside-out, as it were, and then wash your hands. . . . We knew nothing about them until a few years ago, but now we recognize them as Koplik spots." Students should watch for Koplik spots and an abnormal temperature in all their patients. No treatment is necessary, but in children it is especially important to examine the ears every day. Dock told the mother, whose house was full of students, that he would have to report the case. He thought the health officer would not put up a placard. He told the students that "any who are afraid of measles had better not stay. Anybody who stays had better not go to any other clinic today, but spend your time in the open air, get your clothes well aired and wash your hair, then you can go to the surgical clinic."

Perhaps for the same reason Dock had occasion to demonstrate only one case of mumps in eight years, that of a man whose testicles were covered with an ice bag and supported by a board covered with cotton. Dock said that at the first sign of inflammation, elevate the testes. In severe cases, paint the inflamed side with silver nitrate, and the pain will be reduced almost miraculously within half an hour.

Tonsillitis

In January and February students were warned that it is the time of year when they should always examine the throat. Half the nurses in the hospital had sore throats. Dock remarked:

> Every year we have a great many cases, but never so bad as now; there have not been such large tonsils and such horrible looking exudates on them. And the most useful conclusion I can point out is, that everybody has to be careful about his hands and nose and mouth; never put your hands over your mouth or nose or eyes in the hospital and be careful not to blow your nose. It is so easy to get infections that way.

A new patient was brought in, and Dock began to examine his throat.

> Now I will give you a suggestion about that, that you always wash your hands before you put your finger in a patient's mouth. I don't think you can infect such a mouth because it already holds as much infection as it can hold, but it isn't exactly pleasant to see a finger going into your mouth when you know the hand hasn't been washed. Another little detail is to wrap your finger up. Of course in a grown person with reasonable intelligence there is little danger of being bitten; but a child might bite you and for that reason I always like to wrap my finger up. . . . Is a tongue depressor the thing you need most? A doctor must always help himself. When you get to a sick room you mustn't expect the other people waiting around to bring you spoons and things unless you ask for them. Always make yourself master of the situation.

Dock found a tonsil the size of an English walnut, and he asked if there was pus in it. He continued, "If you think there is pus in it your duty is to stick a knife into the tonsil. If in doubt, puncture. The most convenient instrument is a curved bistoury, covering the back two thirds with adhesive plaster, and then jabbing this quickly into two or three places. Of course, theoretically you can cut the carotid, but usually it does not happen."

Erysipelas

Dock said of a patient with chills: "When a patient hasn't pneumonia and isn't likely to have malaria, erysipelas is the disease you should think about." Dock spoke from experience: "In my undergraduate days every surgical case got erysipelas. If a man came in with a compound fracture, he got erysipelas. It was considered part of hospital life." In 1904 the situation in the University Hospital was a little better, and Dock could say erysipelas was becoming a rather rare disease. Nevertheless, cases were referred to Dock's service from surgery and otolaryngology, and patients on his own wards contracted the disease. Dock said:

> It seems she must have been infected from some germs transported through the air, or from some feeding utensil or bed clothes or something else. Personally, I have always been afraid of the sweeping process that goes on in the ward, but no amount of talk on my part can alter that. . . . Although erysipelas is a trifling disease it certainly would be a good thing to sterilize every mattress, etc., with a steam sterilizer if we could find one within a hundred miles; scrub the beds down with bichloride and afterwards wash them with bicarbonate. It might be that some patient in the ward has a stock of erysipelas germs somewhere that has kept up the disease. It certainly seems discreditable for such a disease to go on all the time. . . . If a patient only gets into the ward after he has been into the bathroom, after he has been scrubbed from head to feet, after his clothes have been taken away from him, and after he has been put into a suit that is sterilized and then put in a clean bed, the risk is avoided.

Students were probably not responsible for spreading the disease, but in private practice they would have difficulty explaining that infection had not resulted from their touch.

When Dock wrote the chapter "Erysipelas" in *A System of Practical Medicine*,[2] he said, "the mild nature of most cases of facial erysipelas has made that disease a favorite among those who claim to work miracles in medicine." But the disease can be fatal.

DOCK (reading history): "The patient went to a family having erysipelas two weeks ago Saturday." Always put down dates because a year from now you won't know what "two weeks ago Saturday means." The man in the house had erysipelas, of which he died Tuesday evening. His wife was taken with it on Wednesday. The point I want to make is this; to get a fatal erysipelas is much more dangerous than one that isn't fatal, for people in the vicinity.

Clean the skin with soap and water, and then apply Ichthyol all over the area involved and one inch beyond to stop the spread of infection. Ichthyol was a proprietary sulphonated bitumen from asphalt rich in fish remains, and patients objected to its smell. Another remedy was a soothing ointment of white lead, zinc oxide, and carbolic acid in a vaseline base. Alternatively, the affected area could be washed with gauze saturated with a hot solution of 1:500 bichloride of mercury. "Occasionally you find doctors injecting this to stop the spread. Of course if you inject enough to stop the spread you will very likely kill your patient."

Diphtheria

Late in 1903 a child was transferred to the University Hospital from the Coldwater Hospital for retarded children without a warning that an epidemic of diphtheria was occurring at Coldwater.

In that year there were 3,670 reported cases of diphtheria in Michigan. The 569 deaths came to 22.7 deaths per 100,000 population and 16.5 deaths per 100 cases of diphtheria. There were 23.4 deaths per 100 cases in which antitoxin had not been used, and there were 10.3 deaths per 100 where it had been given.[3]

By December 1st it was clear that the child from Coldwater had diphtheria. Dock had suspected diphtheria before the false membrane appeared, and he had given antitoxin. He told the class:

If any of you broke out within the next few days and didn't have an immunizing dose of antitoxin, it wouldn't look well for any of us. It would look as if we should have coralled you and injected you whether you wanted or not. . . . The antitoxin serum comes at the present time in a very convenient way for using it. It used to come in a bottle, had to be sucked up in a syringe and then injected. Now there is a bulb, as you see, with an end that can be broken off at one end and another one where the needle can be fastened. Over the former end you can put a soft rubber syringe and, in injecting, close this off with the thumb or finger; over the other end an ordinary, sharp hypodermic needle is secured, supposed to be sterilized. The bulbs come in different sizes and with different lables. The most convenient part of the body to operate is on the abdomen. It is very easy to get at in male patients, it is easy to pull up the shirt and get a place that you can clean. In the case of women it requires more time to get the clothing loose there, but it is still easy to inject in the neighborhood of the umbilicus. Pick up the skin and inject the stuff as fast as you can, disperse the little swelling that forms by just working your fingers over it and the operation is done. There are still some people who are skeptical about the efficacy of diphtheria antitoxin. The reason is that they have not used the remedy in sufficient doses, and they don't get any better results than they did with other remedies; perhaps not so good. Hence we use large doses.

On December 4th Dock described a second child who had contracted diphtheria from the first, but he thought the danger of further contagion was over. If more cases were to occur, they should already have appeared. He told the students:

It seems somewhat strange that a child should be sent away from an institution in which there is an epidemic of diphtheria without the people having been told, and it may be that full details of all danger were sent with her. Certainly I would not think it justifiable to let anybody go away from this hospital now without sending word to the place where the patient was going that there was a possibility of diphtheria developing. For example, one patient was to have gone to-day, but will be detained until we are fairly certain that he has no diphtheria, and when he goes, the authorities will be notified of the facts. To do anything else would be morally a very serious wrong, even if it didn't happen to break any particular state law. The next thing is the danger to the rest of the hospital, including every person working in the hospital. The danger of any of us getting the disease is comparatively slight. It is however, one of the most dangerous diseases to doctors and nurses. More doctors and nurses get diphtheria in diphtheria wards than they get measles, or scarlet fever, or smallpox in such wards; yet the risk is not so very great when you have a few cases and can treat them with a certain amount of rigor. Diphtheria is very easily transferred from person to person. You don't get it through the air as smallpox, or scarlet fever or measles, but you get it only by infected stuff from the mucous membrane getting into your own mucous membrane or, rarely, in your skin. But these dangers are comparatively few. In the next few days we won't know how many of the other cases are going to have diphtheria. The danger is lessened by the ordinary precautions that are taken at the present time; that is, the ordinary antiseptic precautions in handling infected material. Those working with the patients must be careful that they don't get their hands directly from handling the patients into their noses or mouths. There is also a certain amount of risk of getting infected directly from the patient by examination. You are looking in the patient's throat; he coughs or sneezes or gags, and a whole cloud of sputum is blown in your face before you can stop. This is the cause of infection in a large number of cases where doctors and nurses are infected. This can be avoided by examining through a pane of glass, so in the case the patient has a paroxysm of coughing or sneezing, the stuff will be thrown on the glass. Discharges from the patient should be burnt. Gargles may be used. By carrying out such precautions as these, we have had several epidemics in this hospital, none of which spread beyond the primary cases. We have never had a student infected; I think never a nurse. In the first place we don't have you seeing the patients as freely as we would like to, because if I took you into the wards and had you see these children as I would like and you got it and others at your boarding houses or rooms might have been exposed to it through you, we would be censured. Here we follow St. Paul's advice and avoid even the appearance of evil. Those of you who are treating other patients in the wards should be very careful to examine their throats as often as you see them because other patients will be likely to break out in the next few days. Look at the throat and if you see anything suspicious in the throat, call the interne and have him see the patient with you. All of you who run the risk of having been infected would do well to take a prophylactic injection of antitoxin. Aside from these precautions, we have done this: We have examined everybody in the hospital who has been exposed to this patient and marked them down as "suspicious." They are being watched and all have received immunizing doses of antitoxin, 250 to 500 units. The nurse has received 500 immunizing units. (Another doctor: She won't take it.) She has to take it; if she doesn't take it we will put another nurse on and send her off and isolate her for four or five days.

On another occasion Dock passed around a specimen sent in by a recent graduate who had taken a swab from the throat of a child with difficult breathing. Without waiting he had given 1,500 units of antitoxin. Dock said he had learned his lesson. The next day the child coughed up a croupous cast of the trachea which was displayed to the class. At another time "Dr. Manwaring, a very well known graduate, who has been carrying out with great thoroughness the accurate methods of work the University tries to instill" had sent an autopsy specimen taken from a patient with Vincent's angina. Dock described it at length and discussed the differential diagnosis. Students, he said,

> must not give up the diagnosis of diphtheria until cultures have been made because they may show that the case is a mixed one, but if cultures and careful examination of smears do not show diphtheria germs then you can easily see the diagnosis should be quite different. Everybody should go over this specimen, in fact go over it very carefully; one can easily overlook fusiform bacilli.

Scarlet Fever

Every year while Dock was at Michigan there were between 3,000 and 7,700 cases of scarlet fever in the state, with a death rate as high as 12.2 per 100,000 population. In October 1899 a local physician had immediately diagnosed scarlet fever in a little girl. The health officer took a different view and refused to placard the house. By the time the girl and her brother were brought to the University Hospital, a large number of persons had been infected. "No one can be blamed for not being able to be sure that the case is scarlet fever but if he fails to take precautions he makes a very serious mistake." The girl and her brother were placed in the isolation ward, and they were soon joined by another child they had infected. Medical students observed the patients through glass, and as a result, Dock said, they saw more of scarlet fever than students in some hospitals that were filled with the disease.

Dock and everyone else took the same precautions as with diphtheria, and no one in the hospital caught scarlet fever from a patient. Dock said that if anyone in a boarding house or rooming house got scarlet fever, "it is quite likely that it will be found that the infection came from some child in the town rather than from you." Osler had written: "Physicians, nurses, and others in contact with the sick may carry the poison to persons at a distance. It is remarkable that in the case of physicians this does not occur more frequently. I know of but one instance in which I carried the contagion of this disease."[4]

The rash, Dock said, consists of red punctate spots separated by areas of white, and the eruptions are not elevated. "If you are too close you hardly notice the white. If you are too far you don't see it." The patient is covered with vaseline, making her more comfortable and reducing risk of infection from the scales. The tongue seen in the first few days is called a strawberry tongue, but a similar tongue is seen in other diseases. Later, when the coating is shed, the surface is rough, looking like a raspberry. Angina is severe, and the tonsils are greatly enlarged and covered with a white exudate. Because the patients had come in late in the disease, Dock did not inject the tonsils with one-half drop of carbolic acid as he ordinarily would have done. There is still danger of contagion when desquamation occurs, and the patient must be kept isolated, perhaps for as long as six weeks. There is no advantage in hurrying desquamation with salicylic acid.

Plague

On April 26, 1901, Dock said he

thought it might be interesting to call your attention to the history of the patient with the plague. I will pass around his chart showing the features of the temperature. The patient is a medical student; age 26; who on the night of April the 4th perhaps it should have been April the 3rd, complained of a loss of appetite and pain in the small of the back, and very severe pain. That evening his temperature was 100; pulse 86; and later in the night the temperature went up to 102.5 and the pulse to 102. He complained of headache. At 4:00 o'clock the next morning he vomited about one pint of bile stained liquid, and later vomited again. The next morning he had difficulty breathing and headache. Just before noon he complained of pain in the right side between the fourth and seventh ribs, from the nipple to the middle axillary line. On account of the fact that the patient had been working with plague cultures, Dr. Novy who saw the man at this time injected 20 c.c. of anti-pest serum subcutaneously. Soon after that the patient began to expectorate a bloody-stained sputum and this sputum inocculated into a guinea pig killed the guinea pig. Later in the evening the patient was brought over here.

Dr. J. G. Cumming, the director of the Pasteur Institute in Novy's department with whom the student had been working, and the student were put in the isolation ward. From then until the student's recovery the two continued to be isolated, and adequate precautions were taken to prevent spread of infection.[5]

Dock continued his description:

About 10:00 o'clock that morning, when I first saw the patient, he then had the appearance on his face such as we are likely to see in severe infectious diseases. The appearance was a good deal like that of the smallpox patient in the fever part of his disease. The face was flushed and the eyes were rather injected, the patient had a somewhat anxious look and at the same time seemed apathetic, and the most striking feature about him was the restlessness. He would lie with his legs drawn up which is rather unusual for a patient with an infectious disease, but one which appears to be common to plague. Many of the old pictures show plague hospitals in which the patients are pictured in the lateral position. Dying or dead ones are usually stretched straight out. It is important to remember that unless a person knew what the patient was doing before he was brought to the hospital, it would hardly occur to anyone that he had bubonic plague. If he came off from a vessel, that would be one of the first things to think of.

From March to December 1900 public health officials in San Francisco observed and diagnosed about twenty-five cases of plague among the Chinese in the city. City officials denied the existence of plague because it would be bad for business, and the coroner was dismissed. State and national officials took another view, and on January 6, 1901, the secretary of the treasury appointed a commission of investigation consisting of Simon Flexner of the University of Pennsylvania, Lewellys Barker of the University of Chicago, and F. G. Novy of the University of Michigan. Between January 27 and February 16, 1901, the commissioners determined beyond doubt that bubonic plague was occurring among the Chinese of San Francisco.[6]

Novy brought plague germs back to Ann Arbor, and he immediately began preparing antiplague serum. He was assisted by the third-year medical student. The student smoked cigarettes, and he rolled his own with rice paper and Bull Durham tobacco. It is likely that he infected himself by way of the cigarettes, and that route would account for the fact that he acquired the pneumonic form. Dock described his clinical course:

The patient's breathing became regular and fairly easy, he complained of pain in the left side of his chest and about the same time he had a nose bleed. During this time the patient was raising sputum that was rather peculiar. The patient would raise without very much difficulty small round masses of rather soft, at the same time, muco-purulent sputum stained with blood. It was not the color of iron rust as we find in croupous pneumonia, it was not prune juice like, but looked rather pinkish, and under the microscope showed large numbers of fresh red blood corpuscles and a large number of germs which to the inexperienced eye would not show anything remarkable, but to the expert were very important. . . . The morning of the fourth day the patient's temperature had reached normal and he was feeling very well. In fact he was so very well that he got up out of bed . . . and then partly dressed himself until finally he was taken with an attack of syncope. The attendant telephoned up to the hospital and Dr. Mattison and I went down then and the man was almost pulseless with a heart beating about 50, and the radial pulse almost impossible to feel, and with great dyspnea. We put the patient on his back and injected strychnine.

The patient was convalescent after the first week in April, but

A convalescent from plague; especially with the pneumonic form, carries around with him for long periods numbers of often virulent germs, so that the convalescent is almost as dangerous as the patient in the early stages of the disease. For that reason Dr. Novy thinks it better to keep the patient here until he has completed the examination of the saliva. Until the examination shows that the spumum is negative it is probably safer to keep the patient over here than to let him go back to the boarding house.

Dock described the treatment:

The patient was treated with a serum prepared in the Pasteur Institute [of the Department of Bacteriology] after the original manner of Yersin. This is a serum that is obtained by injecting toxin into horses and then the horses become more and more resistant, and then finally taking the serum and using it for the purposes of treatment. This is the method that is known to be better than the other method. It is a very expensive method. The horse is very likely to die from the early preparation so there is nothing left to do but to begin the whole thing over again. It has been widely reported in the papers around here that the patient was treated and others here were protected by Haffkine's vaccine.[7] How that got out I do not know. Haffkine's vaccine so far as I know was not used. Haffkine's vaccine is much more easy to make than the horse serum because it can be made simply out of agar cultures. It is a good protective agent if given early. To give a patient that already has suspicious signs is an error because you are likely to give the patient a double dose of toxin. It would not have been safe to use it on the student. Personally, I would have objected very strongly to being injected with that.

The patient did recover and graduate. Years later Cumming met him on a train, in California where he practiced medicine. The student's heart had been damaged, and he had to rest during the day. He died at the age of fifty.

Dock concluded:

> Speaking of danger, it is important to recall that like all rather rare diseases the word plague brings up the unusual feeling of horror in the minds of many people. I do not think there was much alarm here, largely because we kept the thing as quiet as possible so that any alarm that might have been raised had time to die, but at a distance there was a good deal of alarm. It was suggested in other papers that other towns quarantine against Ann Arbor.

Nevertheless, despite Dock's and Novy's precautions, plague did spread, for the plague germs Novy brought to Ann Arbor were later carried to the Caribbean island of St. Hubert, where they killed Leora Arrowsmith. She, like the Michigan medical student, was infected by a contaminated cigarette.[8]

DERMATOLOGY AND SYPHILOLOGY; ARTHRITIS AND GONORRHEA

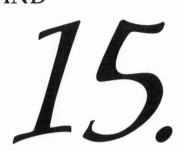

WILLIAM BREAKEY WAS
professor of dermatology and syphilology at Michigan during Dock's time, and consequently Dock's students saw problems of skin disease and syphilis in Dock's medical clinic only when they were incidental to other problems.

Dermatology

Dock frequently began the examination of a patient by saying: "Tell us a little more about his skin." He told his students:

> Every person should know, if he knows anything at all, the common forms of skin disease. The more he knows the better for him. And in order to tell whether [the skin] is healthy you must know the characteristics of a healthy skin. It must fit the body and must not be too slack and it must be elastic. Then a healthy skin has a certain feel, easy to recognize and hard to describe; it must not feel too harsh, not too thin, not too moist and not too dry.

When he gave a detailed description of erythema multiforme, Dock said: "That is a nice thing about skin diseases, the names explain themselves; wherein it is entirely different from internal medicine where we have to spend an endless amount of time to get a name."

A patient referred for evaluation before anesthesia had an eruption on his face and chest: "You can count a dozen in a square inch." Dock said it was not chicken pox or smallpox or syphilis.

260

That is a condition that is looked upon as syphilis among the laity. We know that syphilis can produce various lesions and among them, some like this, but it rarely affects the face and arms without showing itself on the body in other parts. Then the scars resulting from syphilis are not so small and circumscribed as these, but are larger and have a color that is different from this. They look more like the color of a bronze penny.

Dock said the patient had acne rosacea and that it indicates some gastrointestinal disease, and "the treatment of a dilated stomach is somewhat more efficacious in getting this unpleasant affection cured than local treatment."

Dock demonstrated another patient who had, he thought, factitious urticaria, caused, most likely, by some intestinal disturbance or local disease of the gallbladder, kidney, or appendix. He remarked to the class:

When you draw gently with a lead pencil, not enough to make a black mark, you notice first that a white line follows, that does not show much more than on an ordinary skin, but very quickly that white line becomes red. It follows the nail a little more quickly than the pencil, but it becomes red and then a welt raises up so that there is a long, narrow, oedematous looking streak, exactly like the one a whip lash would produce on the skin, and outside of that welt which becomes pale and gets broader, you see a wide zone of erythema. You see where I wrote the word "urticaria," there is a diffise blush all around, but the word stands out.[1]

Dock had the triple response photographed, and he looked for worms in the stool as a possible cause.

Another patient frequently had hives. Dock drew his finger over the skin but failed to raise a wheal. He questioned the patient about food without finding a cause for the hives.

DOCK: Do you ever get them from talking about them?

PATIENT: If I get real nervous.

DOCK: The neurotic condition, after all is only part of it. In order to have hives you must not only have an irritant but also a predisposition.

He told students that calcium chloride, given in large doses of 40 grains three times a day, can be used with great advantage. It had been given on the theory that "hives come from some lack of coagulability of the blood. Whether there is any connection is hard to say."

More often the problem was infestation. A student said spots on a patient's body looked parasitic.

> DOCK: Why?
>
> STUDENT: From the shape of them. Around the edge is the most active process.
>
> DOCK: Well, suggesting what?
>
> STUDENT: Ring worm.
>
> DOCK: Suggesting a little growth spreading out from the center, and happening to show little rings, and the way to settle the diagnosis would be what?
>
> STUDENT: To scrape and analyze microscopically.
>
> DOCK: Suppose we do that.

When the preparation was made:

> It might be some satisfaction to see these things. When you see such an eruption of this ring shaped form it would strike you that it was parasitic and believing it ring worm run over tinea versicolor. . . . Do well people get such things? Well, it is always worth while trying to find out when people have such things whether there isn't some reason for it. People that have them are usually sick; very often they are anemic or else have some condition that makes them sweat too much.

At another time Dock scraped some epithelium, dissolved the epithelial cells with caustic potash, and demonstrated the mycelium and spores of a fungus. Several times he found tinea versicolor, and when the scrapings were examined, he said it is "one of the most common accompaniments of tuberculosis. . . . A thing like that is usually a matter of only a couple of seconds to clear up and then you know something definite. To fall back on the definite diagnosis of tinea versicolor gives relief like a drink of water in a thirsty land."

The spotted appearance of another patient suggested insect bites.

DOCK: Suppose you ask what caused it.

STUDENT (to patient): Will you tell me what caused that?

PATIENT: I was in the Philippines, and had some kind of itch.

DOCK: Dhobie itch, what is common in eastern countries. Did you have it between the legs?

PATIENT: Yes, I had it there.

DOCK: Do you know what dhobie itch is, Carhart? Does anybody know? Are there no Philippine veterans here? Dhobie itch is a parasitic disease they have all around the Orient. It is called dhobie because it comes from washerman. They have washermen there, not washerwomen, and dhobie is the name for them. They get the clothes infected for they often wear their customers' clothes, isn't that right?

PATIENT: Yes.

DOCK: It is not considered out of the way over there in that innocent country. The itch is due to a parasite, to a little ring worm parasite.

In 1904, the year after Dock had attended a medical meeting in Russia, he asked a student:

Mr. Ruby, what do you see?

STUDENT: A hair.

DOCK: What do you think it is? What are they?

STUDENT: The capsule of a parasite.

DOCK: I am glad you recognize them. This is interesting because, while we don't see it very often, it has a good deal of internal medical importance. In the first place it is part of practical hygiene, and in the second place it has diagnostic value in this way: a patient complains of itching without any definite location or any lesion in the skin; he scratches himself and inflammatory lesions appear resembling eczema or enlarged glands, especially in the back of the neck just inside of the border of the hair, and in the hair or on the body you find signs of invasion with pediculus. You find either the enemies themselves, the lice, or you will find in other parts of the body the other genus, the P. pubis. They insert a sucker into the skin and proceed to fill themselves up with blood and the patient then scratches and may give himself a very serious skin lesion. In hospitals it is always important to guard against these things on account of the danger of their spreading. While such things don't usually stay in the bodies of well people who are fairly clean in their habits, they infect the bodies of people who are weak.

Then Dock described the practice at the hospital where he had interned of cleaning each patient on admision.

A patient should not be admitted inside of the hospital until after he has been cleaned. Where there are signs of "life", in addition to other things, a liberal supply of kerosene is beneficial; the patient should then be dressed in hospital clothes and sent into the ward where he belongs. We have not tried to introduce hospital clothes here. They are a great convenience and a very great aid in sanitation in the wards. In hospitals where they are used they have all the male patients dressed in pajamas and the women patients in clothes that resemble the so-called mother hubbard. There is no reason why they should not wear pajamas too, but so far the habit has not spread widely among the female population. They are furnished just as sheets or any bedding. In a well regulated hospital they do not expect a patient to wear his own clothes any more than to furnish his own sheets or coverlet. Then the patient's own clothing is taken away and fumigated. It is done up in a sack, tied up, and sent to a steam sterilizer and thoroughly sterilized. Here we hang them all up together in a well warmed room where the conditions for growth are quite proper, and that helps keep things going. . . . Even in some countries that we look down on a good deal, from a hygienic standpoint they are rather ahead of us. For example, in Russia they have arrangements in every village for disinfecting clothing.

Dock described the Russian village baths and the clothing sterilizers that had been built beside the baths by the army.

Of course it will take a long time to get entirely rid of an infection of that kind; so that travelers in Russia experience an invasion of this kind while traveling in the cars, or even in the hotels, but wise ones protect themselves by a process that I have seen while traveling there. They take two sprays and spray first with herosene. Then to protect themselves against the disagreeable odor of kerosene they turn on a spray with bay rum or cologne water. This will protect them, as I have seen myself, all night.

Diagnosis of Syphilis

In Dock's time at Michigan, diagnosis of syphilis was made from the history and physical examination of the patient. At the beginning of the 1907–1908 academic year, Dock said in discussing a history:

> One thing I would like to point out; there is not enough about the syphilitic infection. One ought to know not merely when it began, and we never speak of it as a sore because that may mean a chancroid as big as a dollar or chancre not more than an eighth of an inch in diameter. We want to know what kind of primary lesion the man had in his own language; try to get the patient to say that so long after the suspected exposure such and such a kind of lesion appeared,—whether an ulcer discharging, where thickened, or shallow; whether there was induration. In that case you would ask, "How did this happen to heal up in a week?" One would think he probably used some specific treatment at the very start. Then the next thing is to find out about the secondaries. What did he have? Sometimes they don't know; sometimes they do and give a vivid description of roseal rash, etc. An internist can never begin too early to know about it and can never know too much because it is the cause of many diseases; so you should learn all you can from these cases whether you get them in the hospital, whether in a steam car, in a smoking car, or on a steamboat, wherever you meet them. In that way you can learn a lot about such things that you might not get in a textbook.

In discussing an outpatient with an aneurysm, Dock said: "A complete history may give lues, hard work and alcohol. The patient admits to two of these, lues and hard work, but not the alcohol."

In the case of women, the childbearing history points to a specific infection. One woman with no history of syphilis had an abortion, two stillbirths, and a weazened, backward child born without hair or nails at seven months. Another with arthritis had been admitted to the gynecological clinic for "poisoned blood." Two or three weeks after marriage there had been eruptions on her face that her physician attributed to ringworm, and this was followed by an abortion and joint trouble.

Sometimes the diagnosis was easy. A traveling saleman's pupils did not react to light, and a little later the student responsible reported that the patient thought he was selling his product to imaginary persons. Old scars might tell the story. Dock said:

> The patient is brought in today not entirely to illustrate his lung condition, but to show the class the condition of his arms, that is, the scars, whitish, regular in outline on both arms, rather symmetrically placed and about the same in intensity on both arms, with more on the right than on the left. If you saw only one you might think of vaccination or in this case of a burn or injections of morphine, yet this lesion here with the history is evidently specific, and yet not really typical because many of them are pigmented and these are not pigmented, you notice.

Another patient with abundant scars on his legs said he had injured himself with an ax while trimming shade trees. Dock questioned him skeptically about those high on the tibia, an unusual place for an accident; they were more likely the result of lues. A child of five had a new growth on her chin and ulcers on her fingers. When a student questioned Dock's diagnosis, he said: "Not possible? You can hardly travel far in this world of sin and sorrow without getting it. Doctors are common victims." The student suggested looking for Hutchinson's teeth, but Dock said the milk teeth would not show the notching.

In April 1908, just before Dock left Michigan, a student said a patient denied syphilitic infection.

> DOCK: Suppose he says tomorrow, "By the way, I forgot all about it; I had a little sore on my penis a number of years ago; the Doctor said it was not a chancre because it wasn't ulcerated; it just looked like a hard piece of skin there and then went away." Then what would you think?

STUDENT: The two diseases may be associated; then I would put him on KI and try to stain for spirochetes.

DOCK: And if you had a dark-light microscope you could watch them unstained. You could see them swimming around in the serum; you could see millions of them. But I dare say the general practitioner will not be called upon to use that microscope in the near future. Do you think you are going to do that when you get out in practice? Have you a microscope?

STUDENT: I haven't one. I am going into a hospital first.

Syphilis as a Complication

Syphilis was most frequently uncovered or suspected as a complication of cardiovascular disease. Once Dock told a long story about a patient who had been operated upon for carcinoma of the liver. A pathologist, not Warthin, had diagnosed tuberculosis on examining the specimen. Dock, however, saw that the lesion was a gumma. Syphilis of the lung, Dock said, is very rare, but it must be kept in mind when making the diagnosis of tuberculosis. When there were central nervous system symptoms, suspicion was sharper. Thus, Dock thought diabetes insipidus, hemiplegia, and complete optic atrophy in one patient could be explained by syphilis. Treatment had had no effect upon the diabetes insipidus or on the eyes, but "there is a certain suggestion of good living about him that is rather questionable, that suggests an over-fed condition, a condition we see in old syphilitic cases." Dock did not discuss an alternative diagnosis, although there may have been one.

Often syphilitic infection accompanied gonorrhea. A student read the history of a man who had come to the medical clinic on account of "awful sickness."

DOCK: Are you through with the syphilitic history?

STUDENT: Yes.

DOCK: That is all he knows about it? He never had a primary sore?

STUDENT: He also states that when he was contemplating marriage the doctor told him he had not had syphilis, but he told him that in order to keep him straight.

DOCK: Does it have that result? When did he have gonorrhea?

STUDENT: Five years before that.

DOCK (to patient): You had the rash soon after you had gonorrhea?

PATIENT: Yes.

DOCK: Well, there is certainly a different scheme; because if he had gonorrhea, he easily could have had a syphilitic infection without knowing it; that is, he could easily have had it inside the urethra, and he never could have noticed the local lesion. Even if he had had a doctor it would have been possible for the doctor not to know it even if he was palpating the urethra, as one should do in such an infection. But if we look out as we should a few weeks after the beginning of the gonorrhea, then we usually find secondary symptoms coming on. . . . Very often the patient is wise enough to ask the doctor whether gonorrhea is all he has, and it is risky to assure the patient that he hasn't anything else, for while the combination is rare it does occur. . . . How soon did he get married?

STUDENT: Five weeks later.

DOCK: And in the meantime he has had no other severe symptoms? What is his marital history?

STUDENT: He has three children. The oldest is 21, and the youngest, (Couldn't hear).

DOCK: And there is no history of abortions?

STUDENT: No.

DOCK: And the children are healthy? The wife is healthy? These are extremely interesting things to hear, but we must not get the idea that because the patient has a healthy wife and healthy children that the patient does not have it.

The patient now has gastric crises and locomotor ataxia. For the gastric crises, the student proposes to "get him under the effects of morphine as soon as possible." The patient is to be referred to Dr. Camp in the neurology clinic, "for, as you have probably heard already, we probably can do a great deal more for tabes than we thought a few years ago."

Treatment of Syphilis

Syphilis was treated in Dr. Breakey's clinic, and Dock agreed with Breakey that there should be no treatment until secondary signs appear. Dock said: "It is better not to treat syphilis until the skin eruption comes out, or you can have a sore throat. You do not lose any time, and you save the trouble and a certain amount of risk in treating a patient for syphilis that does not have syphilis."

An old syphilitic should be treated with postassium iodide. Dock knew that there was dissatisfaction with iodide, "so characteristic of the present time," but "if there is one fact in therapeutics that is well founded it is that certain syphilitic lesions and their symptoms are frequently capable of relief by large amounts of potassium iodide."[2] By large amounts, Dock meant 200 to 500 grains three times a day. Iodism, he said, is seen only with small doses.

When Dock demonstrated a patient with argyria who had been treated with silver nitrate for epilepsy, he told the students that in Germany you could still see men on the street who had turned blue because they had been treated with silver salts for their tabes. When the patient was leaving, Dock said to him: "I am certainly very much obliged to you for coming here. It may be that showing your skin to these young doctors will save some of them from making people blue with silver salts."

A Warning

Dock discussed a patient the students had seen in the gynecological clinic:

She was sent down with a diagnosis of pus tubes and indications for an operation. She was sent to the gynecological clinic with a view to immediate operation, but it was found on examining her under ether that she had no evidence of pus tubes or pelvic infection, but some other kind of infection. It was also evident she had ophthalmia and on account of the history it was thought it might be due to gonococcus often found in other parts of the body, after all the history of the case was based partly on a series of suppositions. The patient married, and not getting along on the most ideal conjugal terms with her spouse he leaves or they separate for a while. He comes back; she gets sick; trouble; absence, return; diplococcus, and so on. The point I want to make is that no matter what troubles people may have and no matter how bad a person's reputation may be, such things are not evidences when we come to diagnoses. We can't say from a series of combinations like this that the patient has gonococcus pus tubes, but we have to find out all the evidence that permit such a thing. Do you get the idea? We must free out minds from all such unessential points as these. It is different from some other conclusions we have to draw, e.g., we find a history of that kind and instead of separation the people live together, the wife has an abortion and no pregnancy after that; in such a case through very long clinical experience the probabilities go to show that there is syphilitic infection somewhere. It is an extremely delicate matter to make diagnoses of this kind, and while one should think about these and while it is legitimate to make them for yourself it is better not to let them get abroad. Always make a diagnosis from the patient and not from the accidental circumstances.

The patient died soon after, a victim of widespread sepsis. Peyton Rous did the autopsy, and Dock described the findings in detail. He concluded by saying: "I mentioned on Tuesday the wrong that might come from making diagnoses from accidental circumstances. The autopsy makes it all the more striking."

Gonorrheal Arthritis

Most cases of gonorrhea seen in the University Hospital were treated in the genitourinary clinic, but some came to Dock's service on account of their arthritis.

A patient who had syphilis ten years before had been treated with mercury and 200 drops of iodide solution three times a day.

DOCK: Well, so much for the history. What is the matter with him now?

STUDENT (reading history): The foot is better; he has rheumatism in the shoulders.

DOCK: The question is, what kind of arthritis has he? Has he rheumatism or has he something else? Has he acute articular rheumatism or chronic following acute or has he some kind of arthritis different from rheumatism, and possibly due to some definite disease, and to start that off has he gonorrhoeal arthritis?

STUDENT: (Couldn't hear.)

DOCK: And if you can get a typical history of acute articular rheumatism fifteen years ago, and if he did not have gonorrhoea at that time or any other disease that would give him arthritis, then you might say that the trouble probably then he had rheumatism, but if he had syphilis and gonorrhoea since—

STUDENT: He had gonorrhoea four months ago and it was cured three months then the rheumatism began.

DOCK: But was it cured or was it one of those interesting cases where "it strikes in", as some patients say, that is, where it leaves the urethra and goes to the epididymus or some joint?

Then Dock gave a long description of how to "milk the seminal vesicle" and identify diplococcus. "This is all internal medicine, not G.U. work. . . . Between the two conditions, so-called articular rheumatism or so-called gonorrhoeal arthritis, the probabilities are of course that he has gonorrhoeal disease, and with his history he may even have some late syphilitic process, he might have tabes, with a tabes joint."

Dock made the diagnosis another way:

Here we have a patient with a suggestive combination, gauze over one eye and a large knee. We think of one particular infection; having given the swelling of the eye and the swelling of the knee, you might by the practice of a little Geometry lay down another point intersecting these two and that would be right because the patient has a gonococcus infection.

Dock showed two patients with gonorrhea the same afternoon. One had had gonorrhea six years before, followed by an acute attack in the joints. A second infection resulted in swelling of the joints with pain and stiffness. A third infection with more joint trouble was treated for eleven months in a sanatorium. Dock remarked:

> There is one thing no amount of physical disability will prevent, and that is a certain class of people from risking infection of that kind. . . . One would think that after people had been infected once, they would abstain from such infection after that; but, as a matter of fact, these people will not abstain from anything of this kind. You might as well know this because if you think you can advise them about this, you may as well know your advice will not be followed.

After the second patient had been examined, a student suggested treatment with potassium iodide. Dock said that is rarely useful; passive motion and hot baths are better.

> Both patients would be good ones to use hot air bath on. Put patients in a machine—get the temperature as high as 300 or 400 degrees. The usual temperature of 250° is high enough. . . . The danger with high temperature is that the draft will start through the machine, even with the greatest care and ignite the cloth fixture.

Arthritis Deformans

Dock examined a patient with arthritis.

> DOCK: How about his bones? Well, he has somewhat symmetrical joints, hasn't he? On both hands we find that his joints are thickened and apparently more thickened from within outward, so that there is a very marked enlargement of the first two joints;

then slight deformity and slight limitation of movement of the other two. In addition to that we find that the phalangeal joints are somewhat limited in their motion, aren't they? Especially the first two fingers, the little finger of the left hand and a good deal in all fingers of the right hand; especially the index. The thumb does not look so deformed, does it? And yet after all we find a good deal of abnormality about the mobility of the joints and also about the feel of them when you manipulate them; for example, as I move the phalangeal joint of the left thumb it feels as if the capsule was too loose, and at the same time there is a certain roughness in the joint; you can wiggle them around, they don't fit; you can feel the condition more than you can demonstrate it. Then we notice the fingers look thin and bony and especially the middle part. The distal phalanges look flattened and broadened; and the question is whether the first two phalanges are not atrophied, so that the patient has symmetrical and quite marked joint affection. . . . What do you think about the feet, Anderson?

STUDENT: They are deformed.

DOCK: But here we have an important thing to consider. Feet are more frequently deformed than hands are. The patient's hands can hardly get in that shape from any worshipping at the shrine of fashion, but if he had worn razor-toed shoes, he could get his feet in that condition. We might ask him about his shoes.

PATIENT: Oh no, it did not come from shoes.

DOCK: So, then we would look a little more closely and see what the change is.

Dock examined toes, ankles, knees, hips, and back with the same thoroughness.

No, the patella is not enlarged, but that is only part of it; These don't feel very much enlarged, but I would like to call your attention to the inside of the patella; on each side the bone is rather distinctly prominent and not only that but it feels rather rough. Feel that and see if that is not so. You notice that it feels uneven, doesn't it? (To patient): Does that hurt?

After Dock removed bandages, he said:

Of course, any bandage will bind after a time, then it should be taken off. Here there was unfortunate economy in using an old bandage. One should use fresh bandages in such a case and use the old ones on less important cases where merely retaining bandages are necessary, or at least not one so old that it is not as hard as a piece of tin as this one is.

Tapping a Joint

Dock removed fluid from a swollen joint, "not only for diagnostic purposes but also therapeutic."

DOCK (to student): Suppose you wash your hands and you might be able to help on the other side. Now you may wonder how you are going to do this when out in the country a couple of months from now, with no skilled assistant of either sex. But very often it is not as difficult there as where you have all the help we have here, without wishing to cast reflections on the help. You have the patient in bed and you go out to the kitchen and get a sauce pan or anything that will hold water and you put your needles in that and your other instruments and set them boiling, and as soon as they begin to boil anything short of tetanus germs will be put out of business, and then you have some hot water all sterilized. Then you take a handful of towels and scrub the patient up, being very liberal with the towels, first using soap and water, then boiled water, throwing away each towel as you use it. You will usually not have any difficulty about getting towels for I never struck a place where they didn't have more towels than we have here in the clinic. Then you wash your own hands and are ready to begin the operation. We now begin in the most likely place. Now if you put your hand where my hand was and push the fluid toward me—what you want to do is to get your hand that it practically pushes all the contents out of the joint. Of course this part of the work in the farm house I am thinking about might be more difficult, but you can nearly always get along some way or the other. (To patient): Does it hurt? I don't want to hurt you.

Treating Rheumatism and Arthritis

Cotton soaked in oil of wintergreen [methyl salicylic acid] was wrapped around swollen joints. "There is only one drawback, and that is that it makes an outrageous smell in the ward." A positive ferric chloride test of fluid removed from a joint showed that some of the salicylate had been absorbed.

On February 13, 1906, the typist spelled the name of a new drug *asperan.* A little later she was able to spell it correctly when Dock asked a student:

Then what would you do?

STUDENT: I would give him aspirin.

DOCK: Why would you give him aspirin?

STUDENT: You want to give him a salicylate.

DOCK: But what is the advantage of giving aspirin?

STUDENT: It is claimed it doesn't have the bad effect on the stomach that the salicylates do.

DOCK: We should remember this; that the same claim has been made about every one of them when new, and although perhaps aspirin seems a little bit safer in that respect than the others, every now and then it fails too.

Dock described the treatment of a patient with painful, swollen joints:

That is a thing we should not forget about arthritis; such a patient should be treated for the possibilities and not merely for what he has now. It may go away, but on the other hand the next thing we know it may be a fully developed case; so he should be treated for rheumatism, put to bed and put on ordinary symptomatic treatment, with light diet, probably a milk diet first, and put under the influence of salicylic acid, just what form is not a matter of very great importance. He should be gotten under the influence and that means not less than 10 grains in 24 hours. If he had a more severe case you would give much larger doses; for example, I have sometimes given patients 30 grains at a dose and every hour as in a severe case we have here where the patient cried even without being handled and the temperature was high. In such a case you can't get the medicine in too fast, and you can't give too much.

Treatment is prolonged. When a student prescribed aspirin and rest for a patient with acute articular rheumatism, Dock asked:

How long do you think he needs rest?

STUDENT: Five weeks.

DOCK: Why do you say five weeks? I think it is better to say you don't know; he may get a chronic rheumatism and may have to be kept in bed for months; then it looks as if you made a bad guess.

Dock agreed with a student that treatment very often will not do much for a patient, and consequently

One of the greatest difficulties is that we cannot pin these people down to continue treatment; they are always thinking they can find somebody with a quack treatment to cure them. . . . [B]ut probably there are few chronic diseases that pay more for the trouble you devote to them than these. While none of them get entirely well, they get so much better that the doctor gets more credit than for one hundred cases of pneumonia or typhoid.

In 1908 Dock described how to treat a patient by making his joints hyperemic. He concluded by saying:

Incidentally I might call attention of those of you who are anxious to part with your wealth to a very useful book on the treatment of such things and a great many others. It is a book on the application of Bier's hyperemia, by Dr. Wm. Meyer and Oscar Schmieden, published by Saunders.[3] Bier's book, while a very good one, is not quite as directly practical as Meyer's and Schmieden. I might also add that the treatment of such cases is one of the most promising things that anybody with a little time can devote himself to. It is surprising to see how much gain a patient can make from persistent treatment, and I have known a few young doctors who have absolutely built up their practice by treatment of an old case of arthritis deformans. If you use a book like that and treat your joint cases and use necessary massage and passive motion you will not make it possible for an osteopathic neighbor to treat all cases of typhoid or scarlet fever, as they do where people give such patients KI for chronic joint disease and coal tar preparations for pain. You can't blame people who are treated thus to go to somebody else, no matter how ignorant and reprehensible he may be, who still does something for them; and then typhoid patients would not have their back broken by osteopathic manipulation or scarlet fever patients have their backs broken, as I have seen done. I hope there are no osteopaths present.

ENDOCRINE
DISORDERS

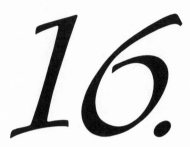

ON OCTOBER 7, 1904, DOCK
presented a middle-aged man with profound asthenia and widespread
pigmentation. He had pigment around the nipples, in the lips and axilla, even on the palms of his hands, and his scrotum was almost black.
A student at once suggested the diagnosis of Addison's disease.

Pigmentation in Addison's Disease

Dock carried the class through a detailed anlaysis of the distribution of
pigment and then through an equally detailed analysis of the nature of
the pigmented areas. He distinguished the distribution of pigment from
that in a patient with vitiligo in whom the skin between the dark spots
was abnormally pale, showing, Dock thought, that pigment had been
lost there. "There is no Caucasian who is so blond normally that his
scrotum is entirely without pigment. So, when a patient has no pigment
on that part of the body, something must have happened to take the pigment away from there."

Dock questioned the students on the differential diagnosis of pigmentation. Because the patient had what looked like "an unusually good
coat of tan," a student asked if it could result from exposure to the
weather. Dock replied:

> That might color his face and hands and neck, but how about the
> nipples, or how about his mouth and genitalia? Exposure to the
> weather does not produce such pigmentation. That has led people
> to diagnose individuals as having Addison's disease when all they

278

had was a combination of sun burn and dirt, sometimes added to that discoloration from flea bites; in other words, the so-called vagabond's disease, where some scrubbing and a few square meals have made the whole condition disappear.

Nor was it an inherited characteristic:

> Looking at his legs, one might suppose that the patient belonged to one of the dark skinned races, like certain Hungarians or Italians, people indiscriminately classed as Dagos; but if you ask the patient if his color has always been this way he will tell you it hasn't.

Arsenic colors the skin brown, but the tint and distribution are different. Dock described the particolored appearance of a patient with arthritis deformans who had been given twenty-seven ounces of arsenic.[1] Neither was it argyria, for that has a more bluish tint. On another occasion Dock presented first a patient with jaundice and then a patient with Addison's disease so that the students could compare the colors. The Addisonian, who had pigmented areola and labia majora, had previously been jaundiced, but her sclera were now clear. Was it possible that the pigment had remained in her skin? Probably not. And: "Over the knees there is discoloration that most likely comes from irritation of being on the knees; very often we can tell the spiritual condition from these things quite as much as whether they have Addison's disease or not."

A Questionable Diagnosis

The patient who had been demonstrated on October 7, 1904, had been in the University Hospital two years before with similar weakness and anemia. He denied having blood in his stool, but on examination Dock found hemorrhoids. The patient had been operated upon, for "it was better to die by the operation than to go ahead and die from the disease." He was treated with arsenic, and he was able to return to work as a traveling salesman for a while.

Hemorrhoids, Dock thought, had been the distinct cause of the original anemia, and he attempted to distinguish between pernicious anemia and Addison's disease as the cause of the continuing anemia and asthenia. The patient collapsed and died seven days later, and Warthin immediately performed an autopsy. His pathological diagnosis agreed with the clinical diagnosis of anemia gravis. Warthin found atrophic gastritis and "simple atrophy and hypoplasia of the adrenal glands." Dock described these findings to the class, and he said: "Mr. Wallace[2] took half of one adrenal and tried it on a rabbit." Dock passed around the kymograph tracing, and students saw "that the injection of the extract caused a great rise in blood pressure showing that the adrenal gland was still active and the patient had at least one adrenal which was active, which shows that the weakness was hardly due to Addison's disease." Dock's conclusion requires explanation. In 1894 Oliver and Schäfer provided the first clue to the pathophysiology of Addison's disease when they demonstrated that the adrenal medulla contains a powerful blood-pressure-raising principle.[3] They tacitly assumed that deficiency of this pressor substance is the cause of Addison's disease, and most of their contemporaries agreed.[4] Because the blood-pressure-raising principle is confined to the medulla and because silver nitrate is turned black by medullary and not by cortical tissue, this idea was called the chromaffin theory of the causation of Addison's disease. Dock, however, had doubts. When, at the end of his time at Michigan, he wrote a long discussion of Addison's disease, he said:

> Not all symptoms can be explained by the chromaffin theory. . . . It is certain that the cortex has a wholly different function from the medulla, but the details are not known. It seems probable that there is an internal secretion, with the power of neutralizing certain toxins, and nutritive and motor stimulating substances. . . . [I]njection of the medullary pressor substance cannot keep alive animals deprived of the glands.[5]

Dock denied his patient had Addison's disease because he assumed the cortex must be active if the medulla is. That assumption is justified by the fact that the most common cause of Addison's disease was tuberculosis of the adrenal glands, which destroyed both cortex and medulla.

Diabetes Mellitus

Many patients with diabetes mellitus came to Dock's medical service, and he told his students:

> When we have an instructive disease like diabetes on hand it would be good for everybody to be reading up on it. When we have a case, one should say to himself "Do I know as much as I would like to know about that?" And then run over it in a textbook, not merely a quiz compend, but a textbook of fair size. I know your answer will be that you have so many quizes and so much work that it is impossible to do that sort of work, but I question whether that is really so; for example, in the time it takes to read what the Board of Athletic Control has done about the Conference you could read what Osler says about diabetes.

Some patients, like a civil engineering student who worked out regularly in the gymnasium, came to the University Hospital because they discovered they were losing weight. Others were referred by a dentist who found something the matter with the gums or by an ophthalmologist who saw cataracts developing. When Dock read the history of a man who had gone to a doctor because his eyes bothered him, he said:

> (reading history): "He has these symptoms [polyuria, polyphagia, polydipsia] six months before consulting a physician." And that is where he made his mistake; and it is one of the most important things in the whole practice of medicine, to let patients understand that when they have important symptoms they ought to see a doctor, and people must realize that there is enough benefit possible in most disease if they go to a doctor. Take the case of appendicitis; twenty-five years ago nobody had it, they all died of inflammation of the bowels. . . . Now everybody knows about appendicitis; everybody that gets a pain in the stomach goes to a doctor, . . . but they don't do it in the case of tuberculosis or diabetes and a number of diseases because they don't understand that the help comes from early treatment.

Suger in the Urine

On November 2, 1900, the student presenting a patient with extreme thirst could think of nothing but kidney disease. He said he would examine the urine for albumin, casts, and its reaction. Another student said he would measure volume and sugar. Then Dock pointed to a table on the blackboard displaying the patient's daily weight, his urine volume, the urine's specific gravity, and the urine's sugar content since October 19. The work had been "done with a good deal of care by Mr. Rich [a fourth-year medical student]." Dock remarked: "It is important to have all the urine that is passed collected at one time. We get the patient a wide mouthed bottle with a piece of paper attached to the side, and 100 c.m.s. marked on it." Dock questioned the first student again:

STUDENT: I cannot recall the normal sp[ecific]. gr[avity].

DOCK: That is the sort of thing one ought not to forget. Suppose you took the normal limit at 1022. Would you say that 1030 is high or not?

STUDENT: I don't know.

DOCK: All these things you are supposed to have studied in physiological chemistry. You are not supposed to wait till you get here for these things.

Dock asked another student:

First, how would you detect the presence of sugar in the urine? Suppose this was next July and a patient came to you with such a history, what would you do?

STUDENT: I would make the fermentation test. I would take a small amount of the urine and put it in a dish of some kind, take some yeast, fill the test tube about one half full of urine, put the yeast in, and if it ferments, the carbon dixoide will expand in the tube and drive the urine out.

DOCK: What would you do for the quantitative test?

STUDENT: I would take the Fehling's solution . . . and boil it, then take an equal amount of the urine and Fehling's solution and heat it up very slowly over the flame to the boiling point, and if there is a glucose there, it will reduce the copper too.

DOCK: Ruby, what do you think of that? Tell us how you make Fehling's.

STUDENT: It is made of two solutions; one of copper sulfate and a solution of Rochelle salts and potassium hydroxide and equal quantities are taken and boiled, and then you add a few drops of urine and you ought to get at that time a red precipitate of copper oxide.[6]

DOCK: That is quite right. What does it show?

STUDENT: That there is something in the urine that causes the reduction.

DOCK: That is a wise answer; the best answer you could possibly give. What might that be?

STUDENT: It might be sugar.

DOCK: This method I find a large number of my friends say they would use, but let me advise you not to work it that way. Experience will show you that about thirty things occur in the urine that can reduce Fehling just about as well as sugar; urea or about 30 other things; far be it from me to ask anybody to remember all the substances that do that. . . . Everybody who examines urine should make other tests, among them Heller's test, which consists in boiling the urine with caustic. You heat the upper part, bring it up to the boiling point, and then if sugar is present, of course it will be burnt. We then get burnt sugar or caromel. On this principle in the lumber regions the lumberman takes caromel, or burnt sugar so as to make brandy, and has a drink that not only looks something like the ordinary article, but produces the same physiological effect. If it is of a canary color there is 1/2 to 1 per cent; amber, 3 to 4 per cent; if it is very dark or even black, it contains from 6 to 10 per cent. . . .

Another test is the phenylhydrazine test. It is very beautiful and I would advise all of you to try it when you get out. The directions are wrong in most books, copied by people who never did it themselves.

Dock asked students to examine a specimen containing phenylglucosa-zone crystals from urine having 4% sugar diluted 1:80. The Fehling test had stopped being positive when the urine was diluted 1:20, and there-fore the phenylhydrazine test is four times more delicate and specific.

James Arneill gave the correct directions in his manual, and Dock would have made the test that way.[7]

After describing other methods, Dock said:

> But none of these are superior to a method which consists in fer-menting the urine and estimating the difference in specific gravity after complete removal of all the sugar; then the difference in the specific gravity by Robert's factor will give us the amount of sugar in per cent. The details of this method are slight but very impor-tant. First you must have an accurate control, and that can be made by taking the specific gravity beforehand and then by taking it afterward but always you must have the same temperature; so the easiest way is to use ordinary bottles because they are cheaper than beakers or flasks, and have one as a control and the other for fermentation. You must always be sure there is no danger of the control fermenting, which is done by always handling it without any danger of yeast contamination. The bottle itself should always be boiled before it is used again. Then the control is kept in one bottle and the other one prepared with some compressed yeast or liquid yeast, the yeast being broken up and dropped into the bot-tle, and then the bottles are stopped either with a loose cork or a bunch of cotton. These two bottles should be kept under similar conditions, that is, the same temperature. Generally they keep in the neighborhood of 30° in an ordinary room. Usually if there is not too much sugar it will be fermented by the next day. Then we make another qualitative test to find out if the sugar is all gone. When the fermentation has caused all the sugar to disappear, then we take the specific gravity of the two substances. For ordinary purposes we can use an ordinary urinometer. Even if we get a cou-ple of degrees off on account of poor graduation the result will not be very much vitiated. Of course you can buy a high priced uri-nometer that will not only be graduated to 20 degrees, and you can get a more accurate [reading] then.

Arneill's manual said that the difference in specific gravity times 0.230 equals the percentage of sugar. In December 1904 Dock said:

> I have here another instrument that is often talked about, but it is not of so much practical importance as one might imagine. This is a polaroscope, and if the section will come and look through it they will see how it' works. This machine costs in the neighborhood of about $25. It works in this way. It divides the field into two colors so that there is a blue field and a red field. If you get the fields exactly alike, then the point at which the index stands indicates the amount of the polarizing substance that is present. If there is 5 per cent of the dextrorotatory substance, then it ought to stand at about 5 degrees to the left. Having the two colors, red and blue, is unfortunate because a number of people are partially red color blind. Otherwise it is a very simple instrument of its kind. The scientific polaroscope costs from $75 to $250, and it is not an instrument that a doctor has any particular call to own. But another aspect of the matter is really more important and that is this: the urine contains not merely dextrorotatory substances but levorotatory substance. So that the polaroscope by itself is not only a difficult and impractical instrument, but may be positively misleading; so that while we frequently work with them here, it is more with the idea of convincing ourselves of their unnecessary nature for any real gain in practical medicine.

At one time Dock compared results obtained with the polaroscope and the fermentation test. One gave 8% and the other 8.5%.

Alimentary Glycosuria

A patient who had been rejected for life insurance on account of sugar in his urine came to the University Hospital to see if he had diabetes. Dock found no sugar in the urine, but on taking the history he discovered that the man ate a great deal of candy. Dock sent him out to buy and eat a quarter of a pound of candy and to save his urine. The man re-

turned with an eight ounce sample containing sugar. The next specimen had no sugar in it. Dock told him to put himself on a diet, to exercise a little, and to go back to the insurance doctor. "The average life
insurance man will say there is a mistake in the former examination
and pass the man."

Dock had trouble with diabetic patients. One patient excreted 150
grams of sugar a day on the hospital diet, but there was no great difference in excretion when carbohydrate was withdrawn. Dock said:

> We cut it down rather gradually, but it was not followed by a re-
> duction in sugar, and the question next comes up whether the pa-
> tient is not getting carbohydrate in some other way. The patient
> declared he was not getting anything else; but it is an interesting
> fact that after having some discussion on that subject the glucose
> fell more rapidly than before. . . . It is remarkable to see how care-
> less patients are. We have had diabetics who were supposed to be
> taking sugar tests who would wander down to the candy shop, buy
> a pound or half a pound and consume that, while we were trying
> to find out how much sugar they would make out of carbohydrate
> and tissues, they were furnishing us with a cheap quantity of glu-
> cose which we could have furnished much cheaper; or a neighbor
> will give them a piece of cake. In this hospital, unfortunately, we
> have no control over such things; in some hospitals the nurse sees
> everything that comes in, usually confiscates it which is probably
> the best thing, and in that way patients cannot be eating things
> that are not good for them or giving their neighbors any. The
> nurses and orderlies should see to those things, and any of you go-
> ing into the wards and seeing such patients as described eating
> chocolates or all-day suckers should inform the nurse or internes
> or myself so that it can be looked into. Such a patient should also
> not be given drastic cathartics so that he can pass his urine
> separately.

Dock told a student to go the diet nurse to get the exact weight of
uncooked food his patient gets, find out how much he eats, and then
from tables and textbook to calculate the calories. Dock continued:
"This is required work, understand, and also it is very valuable work,
but required, just as much as washing out a sinus; first, because it is

good for you, next because it is enjoyable work, and finally because it will count on your record. I mean Karschner too, just as much as you; that is there is plenty of work for two and it ought to be the kind of work one loves."

Treating Diabetes Mellitus

Dock said that in treating diabetes mellitus the first thing is to evaluate the severity of the disease. Watch the patient for a few days while he is on an ordinary diet. Then put him on a diet that is carbohydrate free except for milk. There should be a gradual fall in the urine sugar. Therefore, Dock continued:

> In practice in treating a case of this kind it is necessary to make sugar determinations. Although people do not look upon such neglect as mal-practice, yet from a high moral point of view it really comes quite near that. . . . A patient who can have sugar disappear by putting him on a strict diet after a few days, we say has a mild case. If the patient is eating only meat the patient may secrete over 100 G. of sugar a day, and we call that a severe case. . . . In addition there is another test, and that is with relation to the acetone bodies. We know they come away in certain cases, and if we find these present on a mixed diet we know the patient has an unfavorable outlook in that way. One can also examine the ammonia with the idea of getting an index to the total acid secretion.

In a mild case the urine need be examined only once or twice a year, but in a severe case it should be examined at intervals no longer than two weeks.

An adult with a mild case of diabetes can survive by taking care of himself, by living a regular life, by exercising moderately, and by avoiding mental strain. The diet is particularly important. Find the carbohydrate limit, and make the patient keep within it.

> Experience seems to show that the more pains we take the more thoroughly they can be cured. Von Noorden now claims that he

can remove the sugar altogether from every case of diabetes. I must say I think there are some cases in which it will be difficult to have that happen, but the improvement on dietary treatment is so specific that I am almost ready to say von Noorden is right.

Don't tell the patient to eat all the bread he wants, but show him how much he can stand and allow him that amount, either measuring it roughly or actually weighing it carefully. A slice of bread weighs 20 to 30 grams, and if a patient eats two slices he is taking 25 grams of starch. Bread is best as toast, and there is no difference between white and whole wheat bread. "People generally think they are getting something in whole wheat bread they do not get in anything else. If the patient likes whole wheat bread, let him eat it, but if he doesn't do not torture him with it."

A patient thought gluten bread was made of flour with the starch taken out, and he was eating two loaves a day. Dock showed the class a sample of gluten bread, and he tested the gluten bread and some white bread with iodine. Both gave the same starch reaction. He said the patient is paying anywhere from 15 to 30 cents for what ought to cost 3 cents.

Two very unfortunate results occur from these facts: first, the patient is squandering his money on a most iniquitous set of people; in the next place, he is getting a larger amount of carbohydrate food than he ought for he thinks it will do him good; he is consuming about 200 grams of starch a day, so that instead of sparing his carbohydrate functions he is putting a strain on them all the time.

Although the patient should cut out all sugar, he can eat small quantities of potatoes. Any green vegetable is good, and a student quoted Osler's recommendation of cucumbers. Add fish to the diet, keep the weight up, and take no alcoholic drinks.

Once when Dock questioned a student about details of the diet, the student said he would give the patient skimmed milk because some authors say fat is converted to sugar. Dock replied: "Well, that is very interesting. Fat is about the only thing that is supposed not to be converted into sugar. We urge the patient to take fat in any form, to put butter on everything he eats, to take cream if he wants it, to eat the fatty part of bacon."

When the patient with extreme thirst who had been seen on November 2, 1900, returned to the clinic on February 1, 1901, he said he felt first rate. He reported the details of his diet, and he had kept strict records. He had not eliminated carbohydrate from his diet; there was still some sugar in his urine; but the urine gave no ferric chloride test for diacetic acid. Dock said the man should have a strict test every six months.

If a patient on a strict diet has diacetic acid and acetone in his urine as well as a lot of sugar, give him two grams of sodium bicarbonate every two hours. You do not have to write a prescription for baking soda.

Dock said diabetics usually do not need medicine, but "Many patients spend most of their time going from doctor to doctor asking for prescriptions." In 1905 he told the class:

So in the majority of diabetic cases we see that medicine does not come into use. Here there is a tremendous gain over conditions ten years back. But inasmuch as it is sometimes necessary to carry on treatment it may be well to have some definite ideas about what may be done. In books on treatment of diabetes a large number of drugs will be named but very extensive experience has shown that the opium preparations will do more good than all the others put together, so if we must give a drug an opium preparation is the best one to use. If the patient can afford it, codeine is the best form to give; but the high price of codeine is very often a disadvantage, but laudanum or extract of opium or morphine will do just as much good. The object of using codeine is because it has been known for years that opium has reduced the quantity of sugar and has relieved the nervous symptoms. Another drug is antipyrine and you can give antipyrine for such a purpose without any danger in larger doses than we usually give, . . . although when it was first introduced it was given in much larger doses, 15 gr. at a time. To be sure it killed a great many people and gave them alarming symptoms, turning them blue. . . . We usually give no more than 5 grains, but you can give a diabetic 10 grain doses two or three times a day without any bad effects unless he has an idiosyncracy. These two drugs are enough for anybody to consider as remedies in diabetic treatment, but one should never begin with these drugs with the idea that they are all the patient needs.

Diabetic Coma

The prognosis is poor if the patient is tuberculous as well as diabetic. Dock stated: "The problem comes from the complication; as long as you can't get him entirely free from glycosuria, then you have an unfavorable condition for the tuberculosis. Each is bound to get worse." It is equally bad when dietetic treatment fails or when the patient is a child.

The student following a diabetic patient found that a strict diet did not reduce the sugar in her urine. Daily volume was 6 to 8 liters, and on three successive days there were 193, 293, and 292 grams of sugar in the urine. On Friday the patient was breathing deeply with forced expirations at the rate of 40 to 45 breaths a minute. The student thought coma was coming on. The patient was given 100 grams of sodium bicarbonate a day subcutaneously and by mouth for three days. At the next Tuesday clinic Dock reported that at nine o'clock that morning the nurses had noticed the patient's mind was weak, and the respiratory frequency was only 17. The patient had taken some milk, said something, straightened herself out, made a couple of gurgles, and died. Dock said: "Now it will be worth while calling your attention briefly to the limited amount of knowledge that we have on this intoxication. We really don't know what it is that gives the patient these symptoms." Death is caused by heart failure, respiratory failure, and intoxication. Oxybutyric acid is always excreted in large amounts in the urine, and because it combines with ammonia it does not appear as an acid. In order to overcome acid intoxication, a patient may have to be given as much as 200 grams of sodium bicarbonate a day, but that is seldom successful. Of a later patient Dock said:

> Sometimes you see recommendations to give an alkali subcutaneously. But I would avoid this ever since our experience with a patient of diabetic coma which came on so suddenly that it seemed better to inject the salt immediately under the skin rather than take the time to give it into a vein. So we injected a small quantity. The patient did not live very long, only a few hours after that; the subcutaneous injection caused an enormous sloughing so that the probabilities are that there would have been complete sloughing if she had lived longer. This had nothing to do with the outcome, but the result was a very striking one.

Once when a patient said he had had diabetes as a child, Dock told the class not to believe him. Parents call all sorts of urinary problems, including bed-wetting, "diabetes." If he really had diabetes he would be dead by now. "Patients at a very young age are always from the beginning an unfavorable case; among young patients we include all patients under 25 or 30." They seldom last over six months, and the majority die in diabetic coma.

Simple Goiter

Within a few weeks of arriving in Michigan in 1891 Dock saw more cases of simple goiter than he had seen in several years in Pennsylvania or Texas.[8] Only one Michigan goiter had the grotesque shape commonly seen in Switzerland, and even the largest "would excite little interest in Savoy." Dock went to the copper-mining country in the Upper Peninsula where company physicians had found "fifty well-marked cases in a population of fourteen thousand." Dock surveyed the incidence of goiter throughout the state by visits to doctors and by questionnaires, and he found that the southern counties, "especially the lower two tiers from lake to lake show a large proportion." He reported his personal observations to his students:

> In fact, in this part of the country it may even be said in a sense [that a patient with a small goiter] has no anomaly because from my studies in the gymnasium at certain important functions of the year when people kindly prepare this part of their anatomy for inspection by doctors and others, I have found that 95 per cent. of young girls have swellings like this.

That was on Friday, February 14, 1908. The Junior Hop had been held in the Waterman gymnasium on February 7. Dock continued:

> When Wharton first described the thyroid in the 17th century, the only function he could imagine for it was that God had put it in the neck in order to improve the appearance of the neck which otherwise would have been made up of lines. He looked on it as a

pleasing piece of gallantry on the part of the Creator to make a more beautiful race. This opinion was also held by mediaeval artists because a good many of them painted their women with a slight goitre.[9]

Dock found that goiter develops most frequently in puberty, but no age is exempt. He saw goiter in a mother and her eight children. Those most commonly affected were native to the district, as were goitrous cattle. Horses, Dock found, were more frequently affected than dogs, calves, or lambs, and he once heard a murmur in the goiter of a horse. Michigan has "no glaciers, no deep valleys, no long-continued mists and fogs, no carrying heavy loads on the head, no intermarrying," and Dock could only blame well water that, "according to current knowledge, [contains] the pathogenic substance [that] is supposed to be either a microbe or a toxin." He recommended boiling the water.

Treatment of Simple Goiter

When Dock demonstrated a large goiter, he said:

> This case is similar to hundreds in practice; that is, growing girls from fourteen to sixteen years of age are brought to you for a large goitre. Usually about fourteen the goitre will begin to show itself, and grow in each successive year, the patient being reminded of it because she has to enlarge her collars. Now in that condition old people will say she ought to put such things as amber beads around her neck, and she will put them around the neck and curiously enough the goitre will get smaller and it would have if she had left them off.

This patient had been given "fairly large doses of iodine," and the goiter had gone down an inch. A goitrous neck could be painted with iodine or with red iodide of mercury. Dock said:

> The small quantity taken through the skin or inhaled when the stuff evaporates can relieve the goitre but it is usual to give iodine

internally, as the tincture or as Lugol's solution, 15 drops every other day.

Dock said iodine is rapidly excreted, but the patient

> may get symptoms of iodism that are altogether different from the symptoms we get when giving iodine of potash for ordinary treatment. They are symptoms of thyroidism. The patient has a rapid heart or headache or tremor or other symptoms that we know are more likely to be produced by an overdose of thyroid than iodin as it is taken in large doses.

Dock had treated goitrous patients with dried thyroid, "kindly furnished me by Messrs. Parke, Davis & Co. and Armour Co."[10] One patient had taken five hundred thyroid tablets, but the cases were too few for Dock to draw conclusions.

Dock usually attempted to discover if a goiter was cystic, but he said it is difficult to tell by palpation. "In fact, I have seen one of the most memorable operators make a diagnosis on account of the hardness of the thyroid tumor and when he came to operate the mass suddenly ruptured, and water ran out and there was so little of the tumor left that it could not be dissected out." If Dock found a cyst, he aspirated without an anesthetic, for freezing the skin, he said, gives more pain than puncture with a sharp needle. "Make sure the thing isn't an aneurysm before you go to work, although if it is an aneurysm, you have the consolation of remembering the great Pirogoff made the same mistake." After he had removed 123 cc of light brown fluid from a cyst, Dock said it was entirely a surgical problem; no medication would have any effect on the goiter. However, "The cyst should be emptied and then an attempt should be made by injecting iodoform or some such irritating substance to set up an inflammation."

Myxedema

Dock's informants reported only one case of cretinism in Michigan, and Dock said myxedema is rare. Then one such patient Dock demonstrated in the clinic had a combination of male and female traits in his bones and skin and a mixture of age and infancy about his face. Hair was scanty and had a feminine distribution on the body. The patient hesitated in answering Dock' questions and Dock pointed out

> [s]omething else. When I asked him to put out his tongue he put it out fairly promptly and then let it stay out. It is difficult to keep it in that position for any length of time and we don't often see it in people who are not below average intelligence but we do see it in myxoedema. Sometimes a patient will let his tongue hang out indefinitely, but seeing it only once would be rather risky to say it was a sign of low mentality. He may be only obligingly waiting for us to tell him to withdraw it. Sometimes they seem to talk as if they were wound up and seem determined to finish what they have to say which very often is altogether irrelevant to the question you have asked them. You may, for instance, have asked him to put out his tongue, and after he gets through what he is talking about, out comes the tongue, and you had forgotten you asked him for it.

Dock prescribed thyroid tablets.

Exophthalmic Goiter

Dock said exophthalmic goiter seems to be unusually prevalent in Michigan, and in a typical clinic he presented three patients with the disease. Each patient had an enlarged thyroid gland. Dock began:

> Let's examine her together. We see a tumor that occupies the lower part of the neck, that has a sort of u-shape or horse shoe shape, and when she makes a swallowing motion the thing goes up showing it must be attached to the trachea and larynx. We can see in this particular case there is considerable swelling of the isthmus or middle lobe of the thyroid. That is not always the case, although as a general thing in exophthalmic goitre the thyroid gets large all over, though usually larger on the right side. One expla-

nation of this is that the veins on the right side are more directly exposed to the pressure from the heart. But that is not any more satisfactory than another explanation,—that is, that most people lie on the right side, and blood sinks down in sleep.

When Dock asked a student to differentiate between simple goiter and exophthalmic goiter, the student said there are not many differences. Dock replied:

> Well, to a certain extent you are right . . . because it varies very much in different cases, but the goitre of exophthalmic goitre is likely to be very much more vascular so that it feels like a bunch of blood vessels. . . . The most important thing is to find out whether the vascular changes are marked. We do that by feeling all over, and in some cases are able to bring out very striking signs, I mean a thrill. When we can't get the signs of vascular changes by touch or sight then it is very important to auscult. The murmur must be heard without much pressure, because, of course, you can get a murmur in anybody's neck if you press in the right place with a good deal of force.

Several students said they could not hear a murmur over the thyroid of a patient with exophthalmic goiter. They had taken their hands off the stethoscope.

DOCK: Why did you take your hands off?

STUDENT: Because ausculting the foetal heart you can hear better without.

DOCK: Is that the idea you all had?

STUDENT: Those are the instructions we got. They say the contact of the hands against the bell will make about as much noise as the foetal heart.

DOCK: I should say the man must have a pretty shaky hand. It is only half an hour since I came from ausculting a foetal heart. It was a small foetus, seven months old, freely movable; unless you pressed the stethoscope you could hear, but it was very much easier to hear if you pressed down. I once happened to be in a hotel in a village in this state, and at the next table happened to be a party of doctors. If I had known beforehand I could have made myself known and sat down with them; but they began ridiculing their professors who had told them it was possible to hear the foetal heart sounds. They were men of forty and fifty years of age, and they had never heard a foetal heart sound in their lives, and did not believe those old codgers who taught them obstetrics had ever heard themselves. It was so amusing. I was ashamed afterward to make myself known; yet every layman, who finds himself a prospective father has heard it.

A patient with exophthalmic goiter always has a high heart rate, and in one instance it was 170 to 180. The face was flushed, and Dock demonstrated a capillary pulse. There was a coarse tremor at 5 to 6 per second. Dock passed around something the patient had written to show the effect of the tremor on the patient's handwriting. Dock cautioned the students that there are other causes of tremor; writing a long time, working with the arms, or carrying a heavy load.

The eyes of one patient were only slightly prominent, and Dock said: "When they are not obviously projecting we will tell by drawing a line from the eyebrows to the malar prominence and noting whether the bulb passes beyond that line." On another occasion Dock asked the patient to close her eyes.

> DOCK: Now a lot of illustrious men have had their names given to things on the part of the lids. Do you know, W . . . . . .?
>
> STUDENT: Graefe's sign.
>
> DOCK. What is Graefe's sign?
>
> STUDENT: When the eyeball is moved downwards the upper lid does not follow.

Dock added that there is also absence of winking, and he demonstrated Stellwag's and Moebius's signs. All, he said, had been repeatedly described in the literature. "We call it Basedow's disease, not because he described it first, but because he described it more accurately than any other." Dock taught the students to pronounce Bas-e-do, but occasionally he used Graves's name as well.

The Patient's Mental Condition

Dock questioned a woman with exophthalmic goiter:

> How far back can you remember things here? When did you get back your mind?
>
> PATIENT: I remember laying here and talking about the students and being taken out that door.
>
> DOCK: How long would you say your mind has been all right?
>
> PATIENT: My mind?
>
> DOCK: Are you clear in your mind now?
>
> PATIENT: Oh yes.
>
> DOCK: For how long?
>
> PATIENT: Two weeks.
>
> DOCK: Have you been reading letters for two weeks?
>
> PATIENT: Yes, and Chicago papers and papers from home.
>
> DOCK: What have you been reading in the Chicago papers?
>
> PATIENT: Every paper is full of the Thaw murder case; I won't go into details.
>
> DOCK: But I want to know how much you know. What else have you read?
>
> PATIENT: I have read about a remedy produced in medical institutions for stomach trouble. Mississippi sand is put up in 2-lb. bags, and every time you feel any trouble in your stomach you take a teaspoonful of that sand.
>
> DOCK (to students): What do you say about the advisability of giving a patient with exophthalmic goitre four or five columns of murder trial to read? No hospital patient ought to read such a thing. It might be all right to read the Ann Arbor papers, but to read newspapers like the Chicago papers, especially those for the last couple of weeks, ought to be a thing that no nurse would allow a patient to do, especially one with exophthalmic goitre, a pneumonic or a typhoid convalescent or a person with a serious disease like valvular disease. Perhaps we don't pay enough attention to

such things. I remember some years ago an exciting murder trial took place in Ypsilanti. A typhoid convalescent got hold of the most exciting part of it, the question whether to convict the man or not, and fell dead while reading this thing. . . . I have had the patient talking to bring out her mental condition. When she came she was in a very unstable psychic condition and remained that way for some time. I think it a safe principle for a doctor to have is that all sick people are insane. They are in a condition to make a will; a certain amount of insanity can be expected in a person who makes a will, but it is not positively necessary. Often sick doctors will argue against your treatment; sometimes they will make very radical objections and they are perfectly insane at the time. Now in the case of this patient she talked rationally. Everything she said seemed to hang together, and yet realizing she had a serious disease I took the ground she was non compos. She made statements about the diet. That, to be sure, is a staple article of complaint in hospitals. But the patient made statements to a relative who called on her, and the relative was in great anguish of mind about her and came to see me, and when I told him that what she said was not true was very greatly hurt. He looked on it as a slanderous aspersion of her character, and, when I went on to tell him that the patient was sick and not entirely responsible, although an intelligent man, I had to explain it. (To patient): How does he feel about it now?

PATIENT: I guess he is all right.

Cause of Exophthalmic Goiter

In 1906 Dock said that although the whole picture of exophthalmic goiter is not reproduced by excessive administration of thyroid, "[t]he peculiarities of my clinical material perhaps persuade me in favor of the thyroid as the chief seat of the disease."[11] Nevertheless,

There is good reason for believing exophthalmic goitre requires a certain predisposition, that is, weakness of the nervous system that makes it react more to certain injuries than other people do, and that, in turn, brings on exophthalmic goitre, and how that happens we don't need to go into now. But there are a good many cases that have a history of nervous or psychic disease or nervous disturbances or sometimes a large number with history of exophthalmic goitre in the same family.

Dock also thought "acute infectious diseases affect the thyroid in a toxic and degenerative way, and they may produce an actual thyroiditis."

When Dock showed two women with exophthalmic goiter, he asked a student:

How about the other case?

STUDENT: She has had goitre for 23 years.

DOCK: You think then nothing has happened in the 23 years to bring about this other condition, that is, such a thing as a nervous shock.

STUDENT: Not unless the uterine trouble could have anything to do with it.

DOCK: Do you think it could?

STUDENT: It might; miscarriage and abortion would be a good deal of a shock.

DOCK: That might be true, and yet thousands of women have abortions without bringing on exophthalmic goitre; that is, do you know anything about the thyroid in relation to the uterus that makes you think so?

STUDENT: It enlarges during pregnancy.

DOCK: First, you have striking differences in the incidence of the disease in women and men; four or five to 10 or 20 women have exophthalmic goitre to one man. Here we have found it one to ten. Then the thyroid enlarges very often in pregnancy and very often at other peculiarly feminine periods like menstrual period. But how do you explain the relation between the patient's long-standing goitre and her present symptoms? What makes the difference? She had goitre 23 years and the other symptoms only 12 or 8 years?

STUDENT: I don't know whether an ordinary goitre develops into an exophthalmic goitre or not.

DOCK: Well, why don't you know? Didn't you try to find out? Didn't find anything about primary and secondary goitre? You find exophthalmic goitre sometimes occurs in people who have not had a previous goitre, but it oftener happens in people who have had long standing goitre than those who have not had any at all. But it may be that a patient may not know that the goitre has been there. This is often the case with people who have exophthalmic goitre; so that anybody who imagines in a given case that the thyroid has become enlarged after the tachycardia or palpitations or other symptoms, ought to be very sure that the neck had been seen by somebody capable of forming an accurate opinion of it, because I have seen so many cases of people who thought they had no goitre and yet they had. Then we have to remember the thyroid varies in size from 12 to 15 to 50 to 75 grams in weight; so if 50 grams is the normal, then the one who originally had a 12 gram thyroid who adds, say on to it, 25 or 30 grams had a goitre pathologically speaking, although the gland may not be as large as the average gland. And the anatomical change that occurs in those cases is at present fairly well known. As you are probably aware, the ordinary change in a goitre like this one before the patient got exophthalmic goitre is a hyperplasia of the thyroid all over, with follicles retaining their normal size or else enlarged and very much enlarged so that the patient has large colloid cysts with different kinds of degenerative processes following that. That, however, has nothing to do with the change in exophthalmic goitre. It has been known ever since examinations were made in exophthalmic goitre that any kind of anatomical alteration in the thyroid might be found, and for a long time it was accepted that there was no specific change, that is, that injury of the thyroid had nothing to do with causing it, but was merely an accident. But there is every reason for looking on the condition as being altogether different from that. The characteristic change is one that is well known on account of the enormous number of surgical operations that are made. When it became more common to remove the thyroid and especially in the early stages of the disease, then it was found all such thyroids showed certain anatomical changes that are all alike. They have been compared with the appearance that occurs with the thyroid when part of the gland is removed, we find that a regeneration or hyperplasia occurs in the remaining part of the gland, and this looks very much like that of the foetal thyroid gland. This is spoken of clinically as a Basedow change. They say the goitre has got Basedowized. In the French clinics it is spoken of early as Basedowinian and a case like this a Basedowized change. In that way we would look on exophthalmic goitre as a secondary disease as the result of a condition that comes on as an overworked hyperplasia or as result of a nervous irritation, although in these chemical and physiological days the nervous theory is not held as strongly as it used to be. Most would look on it as a chemical condition due to some altered metabolic condition that required some increased response on the part of the thyroid.

Metabolism in Thyroid Disease

In 1895 Adolph Magnus-Levy, working in von Noorden's Frankfurt clinic, published a short but comprehensive paper in the *Berliner klinische Wochenscrift* describing the fundamental facts of metabolism in thyroid disease. Patients with myxedema have subnormal oxygen consumption and carbon dioxide production. Both are returned to normal by thyroid feeding. Patients with Morbus Basedow have a much higher oxygen consumption and carbon dioxide production than matched controls, and both become normal after either "spontaneous" cure or partial thyroidectomy.[12]

Dock, like Osler,[13] failed to refer to Magnus-Levy's work or to any other contemporary study of metabolism in thyroid disease, and Dock's omission can be attributed to indifference rather than to ignorance. The clue to Dock's indifference is at the end of the chapter, "Diseases of the Thyroid Gland," he contributed to Osler's *Modern Medicine*. After citing changes in nitrogen metabolism that could be detected by urinalysis, Dock wrote: "Kraus suggests that determination of respiratory metabolism (increase in CO_2 and N) by use of the Zuntz-Geppert apparatus may be useful in diagnosis. Fr. Müller observes that this is too complicated."[14] Dock was referring to a long article by Geppert and Zuntz on the control of respiration based on collection and analysis of expired air.[15] He might also have had in mind Zuntz's "Methoden den Gaswechsel zu messen" in Hermann's *Handbuch*[16] or Magnus-Levy's comprehensive "Der Erkrankungen der Schildrüse" in von Noorden's *Handbuch*[17] or its English edition.[18]

The methods used by Magnus-Levy and by Zuntz were indeed complicated, and they were beyond the capabilities of Dock's clinical laboratory. The methods were not beyond the capabilities of Professor Lombard in Michigan's Department of Physiology, less than a half mile away from the University Hospital. When Dock was in Ann Arbor, Lombard, who taught thyroid physiology to medical students, devised a sensitive and accurate method for measuring respiratory exchanges,[19] but Dock and Lombard did not collaborate.

Treatment of Basedow's Disease

A patient with Basedow's disease was treated with absolute bed rest, and one farmer who had recently lost more than seventy pounds said he would just as soon be dead as stay in bed. Dock attempted to control tachycardia by keeping an ice bag, not larger than the size of the heart and containing no more than 3/4 inch of pounded ice, on the heart. In one instance at least the heart rate was brought down to 80–90. Dock chided a nurse when an ice bag was not replaced as soon as the ice had melted. Although Osler recommended veratrum viride, aconite, and strophanthus and had seen benefit from belladonna,[20] Dock thought the side effects of aconite undesirable.

When a patient was nauseated and vomiting, Dock told the students to watch for acetone on the breath. "That is a very important condition. Sometimes it kills people." He described how such a patient had been fed:

This patient was first fed malted milk a drop at a time, and was finally brought around to take food. So the patient was given teaspoon doses every ten minutes; at the same time she had pint enemas by rectum and she retained those. And by the fourth day she had malted milk in quantities from 30 to 50 c.c. every two hours. That is usually one of the surest things to be retained. There is a good deal of latitude in it and the skillful nurse will vary the flavor of it according to the patient's fancy, or rather surprise her by making it taste differently. Then we began with broth and milk instead of malted milk and albumin water, and then she had some tea, cocoa and coffee. When it comes to cocoa, that is rather heavy and not so certain to be retained and so with egg nog. We always mean here a soft drink egg nog; in many hospitals it means an ounce or two of whiskey or brandy.

Osler said well-developed cases of Basedow's disease rarely recover, and after three months' careful treatment one should consider surgery. Because University Hospital records for the period have been destroyed, it is impossible to tell whether Dock's experience was any better. X-irradiation of a patient's thyroid gland was tried with no result other than causing the neck to become pigmented. "When you use x-rays in practice it is very much easier to talk about regulating the rays so as not to affect the skin than to get that state." In 1906, when medical treatment had failed, Dock said arterial ligation and sympathectomy do not give satisfactory results. Partial thyroidectomy might result in myxedema, but that is easy to treat. Those operations, Dock said

are not safe; in fact they are distinctly dangerous. Usually beginning surgeons who have operated on them have lost about half their cases, when they get up to 20 they lose about 30 per cent., and at about 25 they get it down to 10 per cent., and when the number reaches several hundred they get it down to 2 per cent. But there are two or three men in the world who have been able to count their operations by the hundreds.

Kocher in Switzerland operates with cocaine local anesthesia, but Dock said Mayo tells him he prefers general anesthetic.

The patient whose heart rate had come down to 80–90 still had tremor; her exopthalmus was less pronounced; and the brown color of her skin was less striking.

DOCK: I don't want to give you the idea that the patient has made this improvement without anything else being done for her. She had HCl, but the main thing she has had has been thyroidectin, and what is that?

STUDENT: It is serum from a sheep that has had the thyroid taken out.

DOCK: It comes from the serum of thyroidectomized sheep and hence the name thyroidectin. What is the principle of using it? The original idea was something like this: There is a certain antithesis between Basedow's disease and myxoedma. The one has a warm skin, the other cold; one has a quick heart, the other slow. So it was supposed there might be just the opposite condition in the two diseases, that is, that there is something circulating in the blood of the myxoedemata patient that would antagonize something circulating in the blood of the Basedow's case, so the idea was to make an artificial myxoedema patient by taking the thyroid gland out of animals. After six weeks the sheep got a sort of artificial myxoedema; it does not have all the symptoms, but there are changes in the blood that agree pretty closely with those of myxoedema. Sometimes they use the serum; that is what thyroidectin is made of; sometimes the blood. Sometimes they use goats and take out the thyroid, then take a goat giving milk, and then use the milk, which contains the antisubstance. 50 grains three times a day is what she has been getting. . . . At one time when using it, about a year ago, I was more skeptical about it than now. I was doubtful whether a good many results were not due to suggestion because this is a disease in which suggestion plays a large part, But some patients who have been getting along for three years have had this treatment, and I have been led to think it is more useful permanently than I did. Another remedy on the same principle is to make a serum from thyroids of Basedow patients, if you have the material that can undergo surgical exploration, and then to inoculate this into animals and give the serum from those animals. . . . So I would suggest to those who have the opportunities to make experiments from Basedow glands to do so, but be careful you have a serum not too toxic from unknown substances.

ADVICE

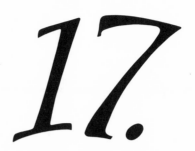

AT THE END OF EACH
academic year Dock gave a lecture on how to set up a practice and how
to get along with colleagues. During the year he frequently gave offhand
advice such as this on curbstone consultation: "Try to be as ready as a
doctor was the other day when a well-to-do individual came up to him
and said, 'What do you do when you have a cold?' 'Oh, I snuffle and
blow my nose, and my eyes run.' The patient saw the point."

Every so often during the year Dock had occasion to give more ex-
tended advice.

DOCK: Miss Bettys, suppose we talk about your case. What had
you made out? What was your diagnosis?

STUDENT: My diagnosis was a secretory motor neurosis, neurosis of the stomach.

Miss Bettys then described the nature of the patient's vomiting and the
pain the patient said she had in the region of the pylorus. Hemoglobin
was 70% and the red cell count 4,300,000, indicating chlorosis.

DOCK: Yes, you could call that a chlorotic condition. As a matter of fact what did she have?

STUDENT: Discovered she was pregnant.

DOCK: This case brings up a number of very important points.
The patient comes with a comparatively common history, a history of gastric symptoms suggesting a neurosis, a mild chlorisis, a
history of irregular menstruation, a whole combination that we
know to be extremely common in girls about the age of twenty. . . .

305

In this case you would make a complete physical examination. So it would be important to examine the patient over the bare abdomen in order to see about that. And while doing that you would be able to examine her mammary glands without exciting any particular thought. You should never give up your investigations in a case until you have settled the cause of the alterations in the mammary glands. The prominence of the glands of Montgomery and the roseola should lead you to examine the internal genitals. One should be careful to neither suggest nor to make an examination without good reason for it. When good reason exists, however, a thorough examination should be made. Now, examining this case one can find in the region of the uterus a mass. This felt from above like a mass the size of a large orange. You might think it was due to a full bladder, and yet if one were accustomed to feel a full bladder one can see that the tumor was too far down to be a distended bladder, and the position and the somewhat hard, boggy feel were suggestive of a uterine tumor, that is, of a physiological tumor. Suppose that the patient had come to you in practice next July, and you found just such conditions, what should you do?

STUDENT: I would make a digital examination.

DOCK: In the hospital people expect to be handled in a more abrupt way, especially as there are no relatives around to have any say in the matter. In private practice one ought to think this: A patient belonging to a respectable family, one should say that the examination of the genitals should not be made without very good reason, and in the case of a man physician without having some member of the family present. In the case of women physicians it seems to me care should be exercised about making such examinations in unmarried women. Suppose you did that and found the girl pregnant, what would you do then?

STUDENT: I should want to be very certain in my own mind before I did anything.

DOCK: What would you do, Lawton?

STUDENT: I should say to the mother that she had some condition in her pelvic organs that, while it was not serious, would need watching, and I would watch farther.

DOCK: That is quite proper. You have to know the mental attitude of the mother. One has to exercise tact about things of that kind. On the other hand, you have to protect yourself. You might throw out some suggestions, as to whether it were not a concealed cause for the sickness, something on the daughter's mind, etc. Then when the truth came out the mother would realize that you knew more than she gave you credit for at first. To finish up this particular case we might suppose that the patient had been malingering from the beginning, that she knew she was pregnant, that she gave us this somewhat difficult history of stomach and uterine symptoms with the object of having herself perhaps sounded or perhaps curetted.

Beginning Practice

Dock began one of his end-of-term lectures by saying: "Now you begin your practical work, the work you have been preparing for these last four years. I dare say that all of you have your minds pretty well made up in regard to the month; signs painted, offices rented, letter heads and prescription blanks ready, so you don't need any further information on those points." Dock did give advice on how to start and conduct a practice and on medical ethics and etiquette,

not because I have an inspired function, like John on the Island of Patmos, but simply observations that I have formed in passing through this vale of tears and may be of assistance to those not so long on the way. . . . There is a large number of reformers going about the country longing to give medical students more work. Some think that what the young doctor needs is a course of lectures on ethics; other lectures on medical history, and so on. . . . There are two camps, the one believing that medical ethics should be gathered into a formal volume and subscribed to as the children of Israel covenanted at Sinai. The other would have every man his own judge of right and wrong.[1]

There are books to be read:

> A good many of the old medical works give very interesting discussions of the duties of a physician to his patients, to his colleagues, to his family, to the public at large, etc. In one of the oldest medical writings we have one of our most concise and at the same time one of the most perfect descriptions of a physician's duties, This is the Hippocratic oath. You will find it in the works of Hippocrates in the library. . . .
>
> In the works of Dr. Benjamin Rush there is a very interesting article on the general duties of a physician, which will be well worth reading also.[2] A book of considerable size has been written on these things, called "The Physician Himself," by Dr. Cathell.[3] It has a good deal of the wisdom of the serpent in it that makes it not altogether wise to recommend to ingenuous youth.

Cathell had written:

> Grow a beard if you look too young.
>
> The best place for an office is in a house on a corner.
>
> Don't use a vaginal speculum as a paper weight on your desk.
>
> Write prescriptions for a woman with suspended menses in plain English so that you won't risk being charged with giving her an abortifacient.

And so on for 335 pages of sententiousness that would make Polonius blush. Students did read the book. There are copies of four editions in the medical library, and their charge cards show they were frequently borrowed.

Obligations to the Patient

Dock said patients have the idea that a doctor is always obliged to pay a call.

> The doctor is not only justified but in fact it is incumbent upon him to refuse calls for certain reasons. In the first place, the doctor

should not take up a patient that he is not pretty confident he can look after. The excuse that he has not time is a very proper one. One should never refuse to go to a patient for a trivial reason. He should not refuse to go because the patient is ill of an uninteresting disease. He should not refuse to go because the patient is a suspected smallpox patient, because they are perhaps afraid for themselves or for their other patients. This is a mistake not of ethics but of policy. A man can then refuse to treat any classes of patients that he chooses, as for instance, venereal diseases. Once having undertaken the care of the case you are not at liberty to give up without some reason, which the patient thoroughly understands, and without having some good person to take care of the patient. Another thing in this connection is the necessity for the physician to do everything he can for the patient. This is a matter that has been thoroughly investigated by the courts. Physicians are not expected to do the impossible, but they are simply obliged to do the best they can. That a physician loses a case does not constitute grounds for mal-practice, but that he does not do everything he ought to do does constitute mal-practice. That means everything with his experience and the present state of knowledge of the medical profession. You should try to take care of every kind of case but only in the proper way. If the patient is a surgical case, and you feel confident of youself, the young man should go ahead and do what he can. For example, it would be proper for the young man to undertake a case of appendicitis or a case of ovarian tumor. I should strongly urge the beginner not to take a case of gallbladder surgery. [Opposite this Dock wrote in the margin: "insist on being ass't at op."] But even there if the patient cannot get the help of a very much more skillful man than yourself it is proper to go ahead and treat the case yourself. In fact, it would be wrong not to do this.

What to Tell the Patient

DOCK: Let me tell you that the less you tell him under those circumstances the better satisfied you and the patient will be. So such a patient does not want a lecture on pathology. As you will very soon find out that a very little information goes a long way in such a case. I found quite by accident that if you told a patient with leukemia that he had "white blood disease" he was quite satisfied.

Thoroughness

DOCK: If you begin by carrying out serious thorough work, you will grow in knowledge, and a large practice will not become more difficult to handle than a smaller one. But if you begin by being careless you will find it more and more difficult to get out of the habit. For example, I have been in the offices of doctors who had no convenient method for examining urine. They told me they had no time, that would do well enough for a hospital. Sometimes I have seen people who began by having patients bring samples of urine, but they never examined them so that they would have thirty or forty bottles about their office. Doctors who work in this way will go backwards and eventually be forced into real estate or worse still, life insurance.

Habits

DOCK: Men who begin to get busy, become hustlers as they call themselves, are sometimes in a few years entirely submerged by the flood and fall back in every way so that they are behind those who are slower. But even those who are overwhelmed can keep up if they have the necessary pluck and endurance. I might add, good habits to withstand temptation, because very often success leads doctors into habits of inebriety that in these days quickly end his usefulness. There was a time when it was thought a drunken doctor was a good thing to have around, but now-a-days people are a little more critical.

Other Doctors

DOCK: Patients will come to you who have been in the hands of another doctor. Many people have the idea that a great deal of ceremony and medical ethics is necessary in such a case. That is not so. A patient has the right to go to any doctor he pleases. Nobody can take that privilege away from a sick man. He has a right to change his mind and very often he has no good explanation for this, yet still he has the right. Many of your patients will be of this kind because they are chronics. Acute cases will come in time, but, in general, the patients who come to a young doctor are those who have tried everybody else, and in despair try the new doctor. It has been laid down that such a patient should not be taken by another doctor unless the patient has been formally discharged by the first doctor and paid his bills. That cannot be carried out practically. . . . Very often a patient will give very good reason for wishing a change.

Criticism of Other Doctors

Dock warned his students that a patient should not be allowed to hear criticism of another doctor who has taken care of him.

Not every patient can be made to get quickly well, and to intimate that what the doctor has been doing before was not the best is certain to react on you for you will get cases that will do badly even according to the best rules of the art. . . . Very often the patient will try to "work" the young doctor in this way. Statements made on the spur of the moment have a great deal to do with the ill feeling that exists in various places, amongst members of the medical profession. And if you think the treatment has not been good do not say anything about it, but so far as possible try to defend the previous treatment. You will find this a useful way of throwing bread upon the waters. There is only one exception to this, and that is where the previous man has been notoriously dishonest as often happens when the man belongs to a sect that claims to have peculiar influence upon disease, such as a Dowieite, a Christian Scientist, and then in such a case state freely your belief in the dishonesty of the person and class. But even then it is well not to say much.

Consultations

DOCK: The question of having a patient who has previously been in the care of another physician, brings up another allied matter of consultations. For a young physician it is extremely important not to get in the habit of refusing [consultations] and very much better to accede at once than to refuse. I know young doctors who with very proper feeling of self-confidence have refused to see other doctors and have said that if people don't like their treatment they could get the other doctor altogether. That is not good policy. You really don't know whether you are so much better than the other doctor after all. You must remember that the other doctor has his friends and influence, and a refusal of that kind is sure to reflect on you. It puts the young doctor in the light of being headstrong and conceited, and although a certain amount is necessary, to carry it too far is a disadvantage. . . . People very often want to have something more done for a patient than is being done. According to the common expression, they think two heads are better than one. Or if a little child is dying of diphtheria or happened to have pneumonia, to say the case is desperate, that you are doing all you can, but to suggest that perhaps they would like to have somebody else, that is very proper, that is all right. Practical experience shows that it is very much better in any case of uncertain or dangerous disease to have someone share the responsibility with you. In serious cases even if they are doing positively badly, even if death seems unavoidable, it is still well to have someone share the responsibility. If people ask you to have someone who is distinctly your inferior in knowledge or skill, I think it is not good to decline. The refusal may be looked on as a criticism of the other physician. If the choice is left to you always try to get the best man you can under the circumstances.

Keeping Records

DOCK: Every doctor should keep records of all his work. You cannot get a more useful aid in the development of your knowledge than in keeping full notes of your practice,—not only medical, but all kinds. If you take notes and keep records you will be more careful in your examination. If you know that you are going to put down a report in your case in black and white, you will be much more likely to look over the patient thoroughly and get out all the signs that are to be obtained than if you don't. A bad note written at the time is better than a good note written after the time.

Dock gave practical instructions:

> So the system should be one possible to carry with you, and the best method is by some arrangement of catalogue cards. Cards can easily be increased in number as you need more and more. I imagine, however, I hear you say, as I have heard some of your predecessors, that it is all very well for me to give you this advice because I don't see many patients. However, although I don't see many patients myself, I happen to know a good many people who do; and some of the men who see the most patients, both in their office and outside, keep up excellent records. They are not giants of strength either but by getting in the habit, and sticking to it they are able to keep notes. They have cards of a size they can carry around.

Dock thought 5-by-8-inch cards the right size, and he preferred blank ones to those with "outlines on them of different parts of the body, the thorax, eyes, nose and such things."

> I began myself as a freshman to try to use abbreviations. The method consists in having a sign for all suffixes and prefixes. Instead of im we used a sort of curve at the beginning. For "ence", which is a very common medical suffix, we would use the letter "e". The same thing would do for "ent" making a different "e"; making a Greek "e" for one and the other for the other. "Con", which is so common in medical terms, we made with "C". Unconscious would take only three strokes with the pen and would take only as much room as two letters.

Dock said it is particularly important to keep notes when you expect to see the patient again.

Let me point out a sordid reason for keeping records. People think that indicates a careful man; if you make notes and let people see that you make them in black and white that will have a good effect upon them. I had a beautiful lesson in that the very day I went to medical school. I happened to get into a car with a young man with whom I was very slightly acquainted, a man who lived in Philadelphia, and he began to tell me about his father's illness and that he had gone to Weir Mitchell and the most remarkable thing about it was that when his father went back to Weir Mitchell after several years, he found Weir Mitchell knew his age and weight before and everything else. . . . Over and over again when I see patients with other doctors, I sometimes have a chance of seeing the bad impression it makes when a doctor says to his patient, "What was it I gave you?" or takes up a bottle of medicine and tastes it right out of the neck of the bottle to refresh his memory.

There is another reason for taking notes:

That is for the purpose of collecting your material and keeping a record of your material and utilizing it not only for your own advantage, but for the advantage of the profession. It must happen to every doctor that he learns a great deal about disease that are either not known at all, or insufficiently known. Only a small part of patients are seen in hospitals, or, if they are, only a certain percentage of chronic diseases. Take angina pectoris. This is a disease that affects largely people of a class which do not come to hospitals; people fairly well to do,—professional people in various professions. It is a disease that has been made known largely by practicing physicians who made careful observations of their cases. . . . Lots of discoveries have been made outside of hospitals in private practice, for example, Basedow, whose name is associated with exophthalmic goitre, not because he was the first one to describe it but because he was one of the best, was a country doctor. Parry, also one of the first to describe exophthalmic goitre, was also not a country doctor exactly, but still living in a provincial city, doing general practice. One need only to point to Jenner as an example of a man who, living in a small country town with a general country practice, riding most of the time, did, of course, epoch-making work in immunity and aside from that made very notable contributions to clinical medicine in other ways.

Money

Dock said a man should never refuse to see a patient who is poor.

A very bright and studious young man, a graduate of this school, settled in a town a few years ago where there was room enough for a good doctor. Some months afterward I was called into the town to see the oldest doctor who was dying with pneumonia. While I was there I saw this young man and as we were walking along the street, he pointed to a man that passed us, "There is an interesting case and nobody is treating him because he has no money." "Why not treat him?" I asked. But he replied he was out for "the stuff", and wasn't going to have anybody sitting around his office unless he had money. It might be supposed that he would have grasped the possibility of the old Doctor's dying and leaving a practice to be distributed.

The young man's practice did not prosper, and he had to leave town. Then Dock repeated the story of the credit a young man had earned by treating a poor woman with arthritis deformans.

While every man should see that he gets his pay, if possible, yet it is not a good thing to put this in the foreground. I was very much interested not long ago in seeing how this works out in a place that is regarded as one of the most highly [blank] places in the country, in the practice of two surgeons who have a very extensive practice in a year. They never speak of a fee before an operation, and never talk business until after the patient is over the operation, and then they arrange the matter on a simple business basis. They find out what the patient is able to pay, but never go to the extent of taking notes or suing people and they told me that they really make more than if they depended upon the methods of some doctors of putting the price in the foreground. . . . Lots of doctors complain about the poor returns of medical practice, but you will find that they really devote not more time to their practice than the drug clerk devotes. In the country some doctors will drive two miles to see a farmer's wife for 50 cents; but if the horse doctor goes the same distance to see a sick sow in the same family, he gets $2.00. Why does the veterinary get $2.00 for treating the sow, while the physician gets only 50 cents for the wife? Because it looks as if more work is being done for the sow. So in case you think the fees are not good enough, the way to improve that is to do more work.

Dispensing Drugs

DOCK: For those of you who are going to practice in the country, strictly speaking, there is nothing to do but to dispense your own stuff; you have no choice in the matter. Those who are going to practice in town where there are drug stores will do well to look at the matter from a broad and general standpoint. It is unfortunately true that the dispensing druggist is getting to be a very rare bird. You can find drug stores today where they don't know the simplest things about the prescribing of drugs; they are simply places for the sale of milk shakes and perfumery and things of that kind. But certainly it cannot be denied that it is better for the doctor not to be dispensing his own medicine if he can get out of it. You can go to the best druggist in the place and tell him you are not going to dispense unless you have to; that you will write prescriptions for the benefit of the patient. But tell him that you expect to stay there and no matter how long it takes you are going to practice medicine as you think is right, and if he will promise to do his part of the work right you will direct patients to get their prescriptions filled by him. There is no suggestion of making any money; it is not a deal that is known as a "rake off."

Hail and Farewell

DOCK: If you follow this course in the first place, acting in a decent and honest way in regard to your patients and colleagues, taking pains in your examinations, keeping careful records, doing careful treatment, you will find that you will get the success that you will all deserve; and if you don't I shall be sorry, but still take a certain grim satisfaction in hearing that you have become real estate agents, writing land contracts, etc.

The End of George Dock at Michigan

In the late spring or early summer of 1908, President Angell wrote to Dock saying he had heard rumors that Dock was thinking of taking a job at Tulane.[4] Michigan would be sorry to lose Dock, but if he were going, would he please make up his mind in a hurry so that Michigan could get on with the task of finding his successor. Michigan was able to work fast, for Albion Walter Hewlett was appointed professor of internal medicine as soon as Dock left. Hewlett had also been taught by Osler, but at Johns Hopkins instead of Pennsylvania. He too had worked in Germany, and in addition to being an accomplished clinician he was a competent scientist.[5] Hewlett left no stenographic record of his teaching.

Dock did go to Tulane. Reuben Peterson said that Dock impulsively accepted Tulane's offer in a fit of pique with Victor Vaughan.[6] Peterson, Dock and other members of the faculty had just defeated one more of Vaughan's efforts to move the clinical years to Detroit in search of a greater patient population. Vaughan had been disingenuous, so Peterson said, and neither Dock nor Peterson trusted Vaughan not to try again. Peterson also said Vaughan had been ungracious when Dock left Michigan and that there was a lack of appreciation of Dock's worth in Ann Arbor. Nevertheless, during the prolonged crisis of 1918–1922 occasioned by Michigan's inability to fill the chair of medicine followed Hewlett's return to Stanford, Vaughan asked Dock if he were interested in returning to Ann Arbor. Dock was not.

Dock had another reason to be disappointed in Michigan. Starting from almost nothing, Dock had built up an adequate clinical laboratory for his department, and it was used by his staff and by medical students performing special studies. Because it was not adequate for routine use, Dock had for years been trying to persuade the university to provide a central clinical laboratory for the hospital. On January 8, 1908, he had written a round-robin letter to the clinical faculty asking for help. Dock wanted a central laboratory in which each fourth-year student could have a desk and a microscope. There should be a laboratory director and a servant to look after equipment and supplies. He did not get the laboratory, but there was one in New Orleans. At that time Tulane was behind Michigan in many respects, but it did have access to the nine-hundred-bed Charity Hospital in which "an excellent teaching laboratory for clinical pathology" had been installed by Dr. C. C. Bass, "who had a remarkable gift for his work."[7] Bass was also a well-trained parasitologist, and within a year he and Dock had written a book on hookworm disease.[8]

The entries on page 748, volume 16, of the *Clinical Notes* read:

Clinic.	Dr. Dock.	Tuesday, May 19, 1908.
	(No report. Miss O. sick.)	
Clinic.	" "	Friday, May 22, 1908.
Clinic.	" "	Tuesday, May 26, 1908.
No clinic.		Friday, May 29, 1908.
	(Examinations.)	

It is a pity there is no transcript of Dock's farewell address, for the last clinic must have been an interesting and instructive session.

Notes

Chapter 1. George Dock and the Medical School

1. There are twenty-two references to George Dock in Cushing, H. The life of Sir William Osler. Oxford: Clarendon Press; 1925.

2. The recruiting of Henry Sewall and his career at Michigan are described in Davenport, H. W. Physiology, 1850–1923; the view from Michigan. Bethesda, MD: American Physiological Society; 1982.

3. The nature of the school is described in detail in Davenport, H. W. Fifty years of medicine at the University of Michigan, 1891–1941; 1986.

4. Cushny's major papers from Michigan are Cushny, A. R. On the action of substances of the digitalis series on the circulation of mammals. J. Exper. Med. 2:213–299; 1897; Wallace, G. B.; Cushny, A. R. On intestinal absorption and the saline cathartics. Am. J. Physiol. 1:411–434; 1898; Cushny, A. R. On saline diuresis. J. Physiol. (Lond.) 28:431–447; 1902; and idem. On the secretion of acid by the kidney. Ibid. 31:188–203; 1904.

5. Cushny, A. R. A textbook of pharmacology and therapeutics. Philadelphia: Lea Brothers and Co.; 1899.

6. Ibid.

7. Wood, H. C.; Remington, J. P.; Stadtler, S. P., eds. The dispensary of the United States of America. 18th ed. Philadelphia: J. B. Lippincott Company; 1899.

8. Dock, G. The university hospital: its past, present, and future. Mich. Alumnus 9:183–192; 1903. It is difficult to reconcile the various estimates of the number of beds, and the number given may be off by ± 20.

Chapter 2. Examining the Patient

1. Dock, G. Outlines for case taking, as used in the medical clinic of the University of Michigan, Ann Arbor, MI: G. Wahr; 1902.

2. Dock, G. Leopold Auenbrugger and the history of percussion. Mich. Alumnus 5:43–49; 1898.

Chapter 3. Cardiovascular Problems

1. Dock, G. Sphygmograms in two cases of bradycardia. Med. News 87:337– 339; 1905.

2. Erlanger, J. Further studies on the physiology of heart block. Am. J. Physiol. 19:160–187; 1906. Dock's comments are in Dock, G. Recent advances in the study of heart disease. Wisconsin Med. J. 6:123–144; 1907–1908.

3. Dock, G. Tricuspid stenosis. Trans. Assoc. Am. Physicians 11:186–194; 1896.

4. Mackenzie, J. The study of the pulse. Edinburgh: Young J. Pentland; 1902.

5. Cushny, A. R.; Matthews, S. A. On the effects of electrical stimulation on the mammalian heart. J. Physiol. (Lond.) 21:213–280; 1897; Cushny, A. R. On the interpretation of pulse tracings. J. Exper. Med. 4:327–347, 1899; and idem. On intermittent pulse. Brit. Med. J. 2:892–894; 1900.

6. Cushny, A. R.; Edmunds, C. W. Paroxysmal irregularity of the heart and auricular fibrillation. In: Bulloch, W., ed. Studies in pathology. Aberdeen: University of Aberdeen; 1906; and idem. Paroxysmal irregularity of the heart and auricular fibrillation. Am. J. Med. Sci. 133:66–77; 1907. The history of Cushny's recognition of auricular fibrillation as a cause of irregular pulse is in Block, M. The earliest correlation of clinical and experimental auricular fibrillation. Am. Heart J. 18:684–691; 1939, in which the patient's hospital record is reproduced.

7. Lewis, T. Evidence of auricular fibrillation treated historically. Brit. Med. J. 1:57–60; 1912.

8. The quotation is from a letter by George Dock's son William to N. D. Munro, reproduced in Munro's paper on Dock read before the Victor C. Vaughan Society of the University of Michigan Medical School on March 12, 1940, and preserved in the Taubman Medical Library.

9. Osler, W. The principles and practice of medicine. 3d ed. New York: D. Appleton and Company; 1898:174.

10. Mackenzie (n. 4), pp. 149, 150.

11. Ibid., pp. 150–153.

12. Dock, G. Endocarditis and intermittent fever. Boston Med. Surg. J. 133:457–461; 1895. The paper reports three cases in which endocarditis had been confused with malaria or tuberculosis, and it describes a postmortem culture made from vegetations on a valve. In another paper (Dock, G. Staphy-

lococcus-aureus infection with endocarditis. New York Med. J. 65:143–147; 1897). Dock described a culture made under the direction of F. G. Novy after A. S. Warthin had performed the autopsy.

13. Osler (n. 9), p. 710: "I was in the habit of enforcing upon my students the etiological lesson by reference to Bacchus and Vulcan at whose shrines a majority of the cases of aortic insufficiency have worshipped, and not a few at those of Mars and Venus."

14. Warthin, A. S. The role of syphilis in the etiology of angina pectoris, coronary arteriosclerosis and thrombosis and of sudden death. Am. Heart J. 6:163–171; 1930. This late paper summarizes evidence collected earlier and opinions formed while Dock was still at Michigan.

15. Henry Sewall had to resign his professorship of physiology at Michigan in 1889 on account of tuberculosis, but he had a long and distinguished career in Denver, Colorado, as an expert on the disease. His opinions were quoted by Dock in the diagnostic clinics.

16. Hall, J. N. Trachial diastolic shock in the diagnosis of aortic aneurysm. Am. J. Med. Sci. 119:10–14; 1900.

17. They were skiagrams, but the transcript always called them skiagraphs.

18. Cook, H. W. Blood pressure determination in general practice; introduction of a practical instrument for routine use. J.A.M.A. 40:1199–1202; 1903. The device was simple, light and compact, but the manometer was easily broken, the mercury was apt to spill, the scale was hard to read, and the interval of graduations was too small. The most serious defect was that the arm band was too narrow, giving readings too high in an adult. Cook was a house officer in pediatrics at Johns Hopkins. The apparatus cost $8.50.

19. Stanton's cuff was 8 cm wide, and the manometer was connected with a metal cistern. Because the relative diameters were 1:1,000, the zero point was very accurate.

20. Janeway, T. C. The clinical study of blood-pressure. New York: D. Appleton and Company; 1904, describes Janeway's and many others' instruments.

21. Erlanger, J. A new instrument for determination of the minimum and maximum blood-pressure in man. Johns Hopkins Hosp. Reports 12:53–110; 1904. Dock's comment, made in reply to a question from a visiting physician, is puzzling, for in 1904 he had compared results obtained with a Cook instrument with those obtained with Erlanger's.

22. Osler (n. 9), p. 774. These sentences are replaced in the 1906 edition by a reference to Janeway's book.

23. Dock, G. Arteriosclerosis of nephritic origin. J.A.M.A. 43:730; 1904.

24. Ibid.

25. Ibid.

26. The skiagraphs are reproduced in the April 1899 issue of the Michi-

gan Alumnus, opposite p. 268, and they may be the first to be published from Michigan.

27. Dock was referring to Moritz, [F]. Eine Methode um beim Röntgenverfahren aus dem Schattenbilde eines Gegenstandes dessen wahre Grösse zu ermitteln (Orthodiagraphie) und die exacte Bestimmung der Herzgrösse nach diesem Verfahrung. Münch. med. Wochenschr. 47:992–996; 1900.

28. Cushny, A. R. A textbook of pharmacology and therapeutics. 4th ed. Philadelphia: Lea Brothers and Co.; 1906.

29. Mackenzie, J. Diseases of the heart. London: Oxford University Press; 1908:267.

30. Doch [sic], G. Some notes on the coronary arteries. Med. Surg. Reporter 75:1–7; 1896.

31. When he was seventy-eight, Dock gave a Frank Billings Lecture (Historical notes on coronary occlusion from Heberden to Osler. J.A.M.A. 113:563–568; 1939) in which he attempted to account for physicians' long neglect of coronary occlusion.

Chapter 4. Diseases of the Lungs, Excluding Tuberculosis

1. Curshmann's spirals are illustrated on p. 154 of Arneill, J. R. Clinical diagnosis and urinalysis. Philadelphia and New York: Lea Brothers and Co.; 1905. This book describes clinical laboratory methods used at Michigan in Dock's time.

2. This and subsequent descriptions of Dock's methods of treating pneumonia are drawn from Dock, G. Pneumonia; the value of internal medication and local external applications. J.A.M.A. 43:1770–1771; 1904.

3. Dock, G. Salicylates in the treatment of pleurisy with effusion. Therap. Gaz. 17:78–82; 1893; and idem. Salicylic acid in pleurisy and other diseases with serous effusion. Trans. Mich. Med. Soc. 19:494–497; 1895.

4. The two major papers are Widal, [F]; Lemierre, [A]. Pathogénie de certains oedèms brightiques: action du chlorure de sodium ingéré. Bull. mem. Soc. méd. hôpit. Paris, 3 s., 20:678–697; 1903; and Achard, Ch. Rétention des chlorures et pathogénie de l'oedème. Ibid., 3 s., 20:980–990; 1903. The journal is now Annales de médecine interne. A letter from Paris ("Dechloration" treatment as practiced in Paris. New York Med. J. 78:849–850; 1903) might have led readers to the French literature. It paraphrased Achard on the theory of edema of Bright's disease: "The salts which are not eliminated accumulate in the tissues and attract the water necessary for their solution; for it is well known that salts, especially chlorides, cannot exist in the organism unless under certain conditions."

Chapter 5. Kidney Trouble

1. Osler, W. The principles and practice of medicine. 6th ed. New York: D. Appleton and Co.; 1906:692–698.

2. There is a short obituary of Arneill by Ward Darley in Ann. Intern. Med. 32:1009; 1950. Arneill was professor of medicine at the University of Denver Medical School from 1903 to 1913, and thereafter an active and highly respected practitioner of medicine in Colorado.

3. Arneill, J. R. Clinical diagnosis and urinalysis. Philadelphia: Lea Brothers and Co.; 1905. Although the book was published after Arneill left Ann Arbor, it is clearly a comprehensive description of methods used at Michigan.

4. "Albuminose" or "albumose" was thought to be a partial digestion product of protein. The patient in whose urine it was found had mollites ostium.

5. Cowie, D. M. The Sudan III stain for tubercle bacillus. New York Med. J. 71:16–17; 1900; idem. A preliminary report on acid-resisting bacilli, with special reference to their occurrence in lower animals. J. Exper. Med. 5:205–214; 1900; and idem. Bacilli which resemble the bacillus turberculosis. Physician and Surgeon 24:8–11;1902.

6. Rowntree, L. G.; Geraghty, J. F. An experimental chemical study of the functional activity of the kidneys by means of phenolsulphonphthalein. J. Pharmacol. Exper. Therap. 1:579–660; 1910. The earlier use of methylene blue and other dyes is described in the long introduction to this paper.

7. Perhaps modern readers need to be told that Dock was referring to Sinclair, U. The jungle. New York: Doubleday, Page and Co.; 1906; a lurid exposé of the meat-packing industry.

8. Osler (n. 1), p. 691.

Chapter 6. Diseases of the Blood

1. Units were never given. The counts are cells per cubic millimeter, and the hemoglobin is a percentage of some unstated standard.

2. Arneill, J. R. Clinical diagnosis and urinalysis. Philadelphia: Lea Brothers and Co.; 1905, gives a detailed account of the methods used at Michigan. The section on examination of the blood begins with a description of dyes and diluting solutions. Frequently used procedures are examining fresh drops, estimating hemoglobin by the Tallqvist or Hammerschlag method, counting red and white cells, typing the cells encountered and identifying malarial parasites. Less frequently used procedures are estimating comparative volume of plasma and corpuscles, estimating the total volume of blood, and estimating time and completion of coagulation.

3. Tallquist [sic], T. W. A practical method of estimating directly the quantity of hemoglobin. St. Paul Med. J. 2:291–294; 1900.

4. The apparatus is described and illustrated by Arneill (n. 2), p. 38, and by Galland G. L.; Goodall, A. The blood. 3d ed. Edinburgh: Green and Son; 1925: 21–22.

5. The last ten words quoted were substituted by Dock for "dismember the foetus when he could not get it out whole." The entire transcript of the lecture is corrected as though Dock meant to publish it.

6. The patients are identified by name, but none of them was demonstrated in the diagnostic clinics.

7. Von Niemeyer, F. A text-book of practical medicine. 3d American ed. New York: D. Appleton and Company; 1870. 2 vols. Humphrey, G. H.; Hackley, C. E., trans. Lehrbuch der speciellen Pathologie und Therapie. 7th ed. rev. 1865.

8. Blaud's pills were a mixture of myrrh, sodium carbonate and iron sulfate, beaten with syrup to form a mass and then divided.

9. This is Charles Franklin Hoover, professor of medicine at Western Reserve University from 1907.

10. See English, P. C. Shock, physiological surgery, and George Washington Crile. Westport, CT: Greenwood Press; 1980.

11. Karl Landsteiner's paper (Ueber Agglutinationerscheinungen normalen menschlichen Blutes. Wien. klin. Wochenschr. 14:1132–1134; 1901) ends with "Endlich sei noch erwähnt, dass die angeführten Beobactungen die wechselnden Folger therapeutische Menschenbluttransfusionen zu erklären gestatten." But no one in Michigan, and it seems elsewhere, had paid any attention by 1908.

12. Dock used the plural *anemias* in his address to the Illinois State Medical Society, May 12, 1902: Dock, G. Pernicious anemias, their diagnosis and treatment. Am. Med. 4:15–19; 1902.

13. Dock was referring to William Hunter, who had published Further investigations regarding the infectious nature and etiology of pernicious anemia (25 cases). Lancet 1:283, 367, 380, 488; 1903; and idem. Oral sepsis as a cause of disease. London: Cassell and Company; 1901. Patients with pernicious anemia had recovered when their mouths were cleaned up by a dentist.

14. Cushny, A. R. A textbook of pharmacology and therapeutics. 4th ed. Philadelphia: Lea Brothers and Co.; 1906:618: "In pernicious anemia arsenic is said to be beneficial, but the improvement is only temporary."

15. Nux vomica is the dried, ripe seed of *Strychnos nux-vomica Linné*, yielding not less than 1.25% strychnine. Fowler's solution is an aqueous solution of potassium arsenite corresponding to 1% arsenic trioxide.

16. A characteristic paper is Dock, G. Morphology of leukemic blood. U. Penn. Med. Mag. 10:329–336; 1897–1898. Dock read this before the Twelfth International Medical Congress in Moscow, September 24, 1897.

17. There is an account of Dorothy Reed in Harvey, A. M. Adventures in medical research. Baltimore: Johns Hopkins University Press; 1974:226–232. She is the Reed of the Reed-Sternberg bodies.

18. Dock, G. Prognosis; its theory and practice. Boston Med. Surg. J. 150:605– 610; 1904. The same address was published in four other journals.

19. Wood, H. C. Therapeutics: its principles and practice. 10th ed. Philadelphia: J. B. Lippincott Company; 1897.

20. Dock, G. Roentgen rays in the treatment of leukemia; a study of reported cases. Am. Med. 8:1083–1087; 1904.

21. Dock, G. Studies on the etiology of malarial infection and the haematozoa of Laveran. Med. News 57:59–65; 1890; idem. Further studies in malarial disease; the parasites and the forms of disease as found in Texas. Ibid. 58:602– 606, 628–634; 1891; and idem. Die Blut-Parasiten der tropischen Malaria-Fieber. Fortschr. d. Med. 11:187–189; 1891; idem. Pernicious malarial fever. Am. J. Med. Sci. 107:379–398; 1894; published after Dock arrived in Michigan, reports a Texas case.

22. Dock's son William in a letter to N. D. Munro, reproduced in Munro's essay for the Victor C. Vaughan Society (see chap. 3, n. 8) wrote:

Historically his [Dock's] most important contributions are his failures. He was and is a good diagnostician and therapist; a sound, patient and not inspiring teacher until one decides to imitate his thorough and broad approach. But as an investigator he was not outstanding. In Galveston he convinced himself mosquitoes were not malaria carriers; at that time the island swarmed with culex and there was no local malaria which came in from down the coast. The difference between culex and anopheles came later and explained this error.

I have pestered authorities on the history of malaria, but I have been unable to find any other statement of this error.

23. Dock, G. Mosquitoes and malaria; the present knowledge of their relations, with some observations in Ann Arbor and vicinity. Mich. State Med. J. 2:37–45; 1903.

24. See Smith, D. C. The rise and fall of typho-malarial fever. J. Hist. Med. 37:182–220, 287–321; 1982.

25. Dock, G. Quinine in malaria. J.A.M.A. 33:248–253; 1899.

Chapter 7. Ascites

1. The reference in Dock's handwriting is so illegible that I have been unable to identify it.

2. Dock twice published a full case history: Dock, G. Chylous ascites and chylous pleurisy, in a case of lymphocytoma involving the thoracic duct. Am. J. Med. Sci. 134:634–643; 1907; and idem. Chylous ascites. Trans. Assoc. Am. Physicians 22:464–476; 1907.

3. Dock, G. A plea for laparotomy rather than paracentesis in ascites. Internat. Clin., 17th ser., 2:51–63; 1907.

Chapter 8. Mouth, Esophagus and Stomach

1. Dock, G. The diagnosis of obstruction of the oesophagus. J. Mich. Med. Soc. 7:435–439; 1908.

2. Osler, W. The principles and practice of medicine. 6th ed. New York. D. Appleton and Co.; 1906:453.

3. This patient is described more fully in Dock, G.; Warthin, A. S. A clinical and pathological study of two cases of splenic anemia, with early and late stages of cirrhosis. Am. J. Med. Sci. 127:24–55; 1904.

4. David Murray Cowie made extensive studies of gastric secretion while he was Dock's assistant between 1896 and 1903. See Cowie, D. M. Hyperacidity of stomach contents. Physician and Surgeon 23:400–411; 1901; and Cowie, D. M.; Inch, F. A. Clinical investigation of the digestion in the insane. Am. J. Med. Sci. 130:460–492; 1905. The latter study was based on the assumption that if neurotic patients have disordered gastric secretion, then certified insane patients should have really abnormal gastric function. Cowie and Inch, the latter a physician at the Kalamazoo State Hospital for the Insane, found very little difference.

5. Novy, F. G. Laboratory work in physiological chemistry. Ann Arbor: George Wahr; 1898.

6. Dock, G. Methods, values and limitations of the knowledge of gastric contents. J.A.M.A. 45:1385–1387; 1905.

7. Osler (n. 2), 3d ed., 1898, p. 543.

8. Pavlov, I. P. The work of the digestive glands. London: Charles Griffin and Company; 1902. Thompson, W. H., trans. Die Arbeit der Verdauungsdrüsen. 1902.

9. Cowie, D. M.; Munson, J. F. An experimental study of the action of oil on gastric acidity and motility. Arch. Intern. Med. 1:61–101; 1898. Munson had been an instructor at Michigan, and he did a parallel study at the Craig Colony, Sonyea, NY, using cottonseed oil.

10. Dock, G. Medical considerations of gastric surgery. Yale Med. J. 11:359–382; 1904–1905.

Chapter 9. The Lower Digestive Tract

1. Kelly's proctoscope is described and illustrated on p. 41 of Kelly, H. A. Gynecological technic. In: Kelly, H. A.; Noble, C. P., eds. Gynecology and abdominal surgery. Philadelphia: W. B. Saunders Company; 1907. It was a metal tube 18 cm long and 2.1 cm inside diameter, and it had a pistol-grip handle. An obturator with a parabolic end was removed after the instrument had been inserted.

2. See the entry on witch hazel in Brunton, T. L. A text-book of pharmacology, therapeutics and materia medica. Adapted to the United States pharmacopoeia by Williams, F. H. 3d ed. Philadelphia: Lea Brothers and Co.; 1889:1029.

3. Dock, G. Appendicitis, etiology, pathology and clinical course. Clin. Rev. 12:411–418; 1900.

4. Only one patient with amoebic dysentery was not a Spanish War veteran. That patient was presented in the clinic on December 10, 1901, and described in Dock, G. Amebic dysentery in Michigan. J.A.M.A. 39:617–620; 1902. Dock justified the report on account of the geographical distribution; the patient had never been out of Michigan except to Chicago in 1893. Reddish brown mucus had been collected at the first rectal examination, and on microscopic examination Dock saw several large amoebas and Charcot's crystals. Dock included in his paper a long review of the opinions of those who thought amoebas are normal commensals in the human intestine. He said he had given Carlsbad salts [sodium bicarbonate and sulfate] to all patients with no contraindications and had examined more than 200 stools, finding flagellates but no amoebas except in one caes of ulcerated cancer of the rectum. The number 200 may be in the same mathematical class as Dock's "many thousands" of gastric analyses.

5. Dock, G. Animal parasites. In: Loomis, A. L.; Thompson, W. G., eds. A system of practical medicine. Philadelphia: Lea Brothers and Co.; 1898; 2:315–349.

6. See Brunton (n. 2), p. 1066, and Cushny, A. R. A textbook of pharmacology and therapeutics. 4th ed. Philadelphia: Lea Brothers and Co.; 1906: 1066. Male fern is an ethereal extract of the rhyzomes with persistent bases of the petioles of *Aspidistra filix* mas. Its active ingredient was thought to be filicic acid, but Cushny thought there were others as well.

Chapter 10. Gallbladder and Gallstones

1. Stokes, W. Lectures on the theory and practice of medicine; lecture XII: on jaundice. Lond. Med. Surg. J. 5:197–201; 1839. The quotation continues

with Stokes's emphasis: "Inflammation of the upper part of the digestive tube is an extremely frequent cause of jaundice, and this result is, generally speaking, *independent of any mechanical obstruction of the gall bladder or biliary ducts.*"

2. Virchow, R. Ueber das Vorkommen und den Nachweis des hepatogen, inbesonders des katarrhalischer Icterus. Arch. f. path. Anat. u. Physiol. 33:117–125; 1865.

3. Osler, W. The principles and practice of medicine. 3d ed. New York: D. Appleton and Company; 1896:555. A fuller quotation is

The catarrhal condition now under consideration is probably always an extension of gastro-duodenal catarrh, and the process is most intense in the *pars intestinalis* of the duct, which projects into the duodenum. . . . It is not known how widespread this catarrh is in the bile passages, and whether it really passes up the ducts. . . . This catarrh or simple jaundice results from the following causes: (1) Duodenual catarrh in whatever way produced, most commonly following attacks of indigestion.

The 1906 edition is similar.

4. Dock, G. Medical treatment of cholelithiasis. J.A.M.A. 49:1414–1416; 1907.

5. Peterson, R. Gall-stones during the course of 1,066 abdominal sections for pelvic disease. Surg. Gynecol. Obstet. 20:284–291; 1915.

6. Kehr, H. Anleitung zur Erlehrnung der Diagnostik der einzelenen Formen der Gallsteinenkrankheit, auf Grund eigener, bei 433 Gallsteinopertationen. Berlin: Verlag von Fischers Medicinischer Buchhandlung; 1899:118–119.

Chapter 11. Infectious Diseases: Typhoid Fever

1. Reed, W.; Vaughan, V. C.; Shakespeare, E. O. Report on the origin and spread of typhoid fever in the U.S. military camps during the Spanish War of 1898. 2 vols. Washington, D.C.: Government Printing Office; 1904. Dock's views on the diagnosis of typhoid fever are in Dock, G. Typho-malarial fever, so-called. New York Med. J. 69:253–258; 1899.

2. Ibid., pp. 677ff.

3. Annual report of the secretary of the State Board of Health of the state of Michigan for the fiscal year ending June 30, 1908. Lansing, MI: Robert Smith Printing Co.; 1908.

4. Dock, G. Diet and medicine in the treatment of typhoid fever in the Uni-

versity Hospital, Ann Arbor, Michigan. Physician and Surgeon 30:481–485; 1908.

5. Curshmann, H. Typhoid fever and typhus fever. Osler, W., ed. Philadelphia: W. B. Saunders and Co.; 1900:305–309.

6. Osler, W. The principle and practice of medicine. 6th ed. New York: D. Appleton and Co.; 1906:71.

7. Curshmann (n. 5), p. 113.

8. Widal, F. Serodiagnostic de fièvre typhoid. Bull. mem. Soc. méd. hôpit. Paris, 3 s., 13:561–566; 1896.

9. Arneill, J. R. Clinical diagnosis and urinalysis. Philadelphia: Lea Brothers and Co.; 1905:64–67.

10. This is republished in part in Collected papers of Paul Ehrlich. vol. 1. London: Pergamon Press; 1976:619–629. I have not seen the original publication.

11. Osler (n. 6), p. 87.

12. Ibid., pp. 101–102.

13. Dock (n. 4).

14. Osler (n. 6), pp. 77, 851.

15. This is Duncan Lorne Alexander, M:D., Michigan 1903, intern in internal medicine at the University Hospital.

Chapter 12. Infectious Diseases: Tuberculosis

1. Annual report of the secretary of the State Board of Health of the state of Michigan for the fiscal year ending June 30, 1908. Lansing, MI: Robert Smith Printing Co.; 1908.

2. Dock, G.; Chadbourne, T. L. An etiologic study of tuberculosis in country people. Phila. Med. J. 2:966–970; 1898. Chadbourne had been a demonstrator on Dock's service.

3. Ibid.

4. Ibid.

5. Ibid.

6. There is nothing in the transcript relating what happened to the other seven patients.

7. Cowie, D. M. The Sudan III stain for tubercle cacillus. New York Med. J. 71:16–17; 1900; and idem. A preliminary report on acid-resisting bacilli, with special reference to their occurrence in lower animals. J. Exper. Med. 5:205–214; 1900.

8. See Wright, A. E. Studies on immunization. New York: William Wood

and Company; 1910. This consists largely of reprints of earlier papers that would have been seen by Dock at the time of their publication. The definition of the opsonic index is

> Blood fluids modify the bacteria in a manner which renders them a ready prey to the phagocytes. We may speak of this as an "opsonic" effect (opsonos—I cater for; I prepare victuals for), and we may use the term "opsonins" to designate the elements in the blood which produce this effect. . . . [The index is the] ratio in which the phagocytic power of the patient's blood stood in each case to the phagocytic or opsonic power of the normal individual who furnishes the control blood.

9. Annual report (n. 1).

10. Dock was referring to Goetsch. Ueber die Behandlung der Lungentuberkulose mit Tuberkulin. Dtsch. med. Wochenshr. 27:405–410; 1901. The author was Geh. San.-Path., and like other similarly exalted persons, he did not use a first initial.

11. I have not identified the quotation in Holmes's writings. The next sentence refers to the fact that Richard Cabot lectured on philosophy at Harvard College.

12. Vaughan, V. C. The nucleins and nuclein therapy. J.A.M.A. 22:823–831; 1894; and idem. The treatment of tuberculosis with yeast-nuclein. Med. News 65:657–659, 675–681; 1894.

13. Dock, G. Some reasons why there should be a hospital for consumptives in connection with the University Hospital. Physician and Surgeon 24:60–65; 1902.

14. Despite Dock's explanation quoted below, I use *sanatorium*, and I have substituted it for the randomly distributed *sanitarium* in the Clinical Notes. The typist used both spellings.

15. This is Jabez H. Elliott, M.D., Toronto 1897, and the institution was the Muskoka Free Hospital for Consumptives, est. 1902.

Chapter 13. Smallpox

1. Small pox, small-pox, and smallpox are used interchangeably in the typescript. I have changed the first two to the last throughout.

2. Annual report of the secretary of the State Board of Health of the state of Michigan for the fiscal year ending June 30, 1908. Lansing, MI: Robert Smith Printing Co.; 1908.

3. Dock, G. Compulsory vaccination, antivaccination, and organized vaccination. Am. J. Med. Sci. 133:218–233; 1907. This contains a long review of laws and tort cases relating to vaccination.

4. Shaw, W. B., ed. The University of Michigan, an encyclopedic survey. Ann Arbor: University of Michigan Press; 1942:1657.

5. The English version is Kaposi, M. Pathology and treatment of diseases of the skin. New York: W. Wood and Company; 1895:177. Johnston, J. C., trans. Pathologie und Therapie der Hautkrankheiten. Wien und Leipzig: Urban & Schwartzenberg; 1893: "I cannot enter into details, but I recognize only a single form of variola, derived from a single virus, which may occur with more or less severe, even fatal symptoms, and at other times runs its course as an insignificant disease. With Hebra I regard it as practicable to recognize three classes of variola, according to their severity—viz., variola vera, varioloid, and varicella."

6. Dock, G. Printed editions of the Rosa Anglica of John of Gaddesden. Janus 12:425–435; 1907; records Dock's correspondence with many librarians in Europe to determine their holdings of the 1492 and subsequent editions. Dock's own copy was the Venice 1502 edition. His translation of the crucial passage is, "Let scarlet be taken and let him who is suffering from smallpox be entirely wrapped in it or in some other red cloth. Thus I did when the son of the illustrious King of England suffered from smallpox. I took care that everything about the couch should be red and his cure was perfectly effected, for he was restored to health without a trace of the pocks."

See also Chomley, H. P. John of Gaddesden and the rosa medicinae. Oxford: Clarendon Press; 1912. Because John of Gaddesden lived early in the fourteenth century and Chaucer late in the same century, and because they were both connected with the royal court, some have asserted that Chaucer's Doctour of Phisike is modeled on John. Dock's article begins with a long quotation from the *Canterbury Tales*.

7. The English version is Finsen, N. R. Phototherapy. London: Edward Arnold; 1901. Sequera, J. H., trans. Ueber die Bedeutung der chemischen Strahlen des Lichtes für Medicin und Biologie. Leipzig: F. C. W. Vogel; 1899.

8. It is remotely possible that Dock's supposition that medical students frequented Bible classes is ironical. Alice Hamilton was disturbed by Dock's "sarcastic remarks about religion." See Sicherman, B. Alice Hamilton, a life in letters. Cambridge: Harvard University Press; 1984:42.

9. Dock (n. 3).

10. Dock, G. Vaccination. In: Osler, W., ed. Modern medicine. Philadelphia: Lea Brothers and Co.; 1907; 3:301–328.

11. Dock, G. Smallpox and vaccination with special reference to glycerinated lymph. J.A.M.A. 37:1677–1679; 1901.

Chapter 14. More Infectious Diseases

1. Annual report of the secretary of the State Board of Health of the state of Michigan for the fiscal year ending June 30, 1908. Lansing, MI: Robert Smith Printing Co.; 1908.

2. Dock, G. Erysipelas. In: Loomis, A. L.; Thompson, W. G., eds. A system of practical medicine. New York: Lea Brothers and Co.; 1897–1898; 1 451–475.

3. Annual report (n. 1).

4. Osler, W. The principles and practice of medicine. 3d ed. New York: D. Appleton and Company; 1896:76.

5. The plague story is a splendid example of the unreliability of testimony of participants. Cumming, in an article published sixty years after the event, said the student became ill on June 1, 1901. See Cumming, J. G. The plague, a laboratory case report. Military Med. 128:435–439; 1963. Cumming said Barker was professor of clinical medicine at Johns Hopkins at the time, but Barker was professor of anatomy at Chicago. Details of isolation of the student and Cumming and Cumming's meeting with the student many years later may be correct. Victor Vaughan once said that the student had stolen the culture, but other testimony is that the student was working in the laboratory preparing a vaccine. Because the Clinical Notes are a primary document, I follow Dock rather than Cumming or Vaughan.

6. Flexner, S.; Novy, F. G.; Barker, L. F. Report of the commission appointed by the secretary of the treasury for the investigation of plague in San Francisco, under instruction from the surgeon-general, Marine Hospital Service. Washington, D.C.: Government Printing Office; 1901.

7. See Haffkine, W. M. Remarks on the plague prophylactic fluid. Brit. Med. J. 1:1461–1462; 1897. Haffkine's vaccine was not made on agar but on ghee floating on a culture medium.

8. Sinclair Lewis, as is well known, got his bacteriological and medical information from Paul DeKruif, who had been Novy's student for many years. See Schorer, M. Sinclair Lewis, an American life. New York: McGraw-Hill Book Company; 1961.

Chapter 15. Dermatology and Syphilology; Arthritis and Gonorrhea

1. Sir Thomas Lewis said factitious urticaria "has been regarded generally as pathological, and has been associated, unguardedly and erroneously with distinct diseases too numerous to name." See Lewis, T. The blood vessels of the human skin and their responses. London: Shaw and Sons; 1927:11.

2. Dock, G. The advantage of using potassium iodide until we have something better. J.A.M.A. 53:1607–1608; 1909.

3. Dock was referring to Meyer, W.; Schmieden, V. Bier's hyperemic treatment in surgery, medicine, and the specialties; a manual of its practical application. Philadelphia: W. B. Saunders Company; 1908. The copy in the Taubman Medical Library is inscribed "Department of Internal Medicine" in Dock's hand, and its price was $3.00. Meyer was Willy Meyer, the immigrant surgeon practicing in New York, and Schmieden was Bier's assistant at the University of Berlin. The book was derived from Bier, A. K. G. Hyperämie als Heilmittel, 4th ed. Leipzig: F. C. W. Vogel; 1906. The English edition, obviously the one referred to by Dock, is far more liberally illustrated than the German volume on which it is based.

Chapter 16. Endocrine Disorders

1. Alexander, D. L. A case of arthritis deformans in which large doses of arsenic were taken. J.A.M.A. 44:627–629; 1905. Alexander was an intern on Dock's service.

2. This is George B. Wallace, M.D., Michigan 1897, instructor in pharmacology and Arthur Cushny's collaborator in demonstrating the mechanism of saline catharsis. Wallace was later professor of pharmacology at New York University for many years.

3. Oliver, G.; Schäfer, E. A. On the physiological action of extract of the suprarenal capsules. J. Physiol. (Lond.) 16:1–4; 1894; and 17:9–14; 1895. These abstracts are the summary of the full-dress paper published in J. Physiol. (Lond.) 18:230–279; 1895.

4. For a detailed analysis of the reasons for this belief, see Wilson, L. G. Internal secretions in disease: the historical relation of clinical medicine and scientific physiology. J. Hist. Med. 39:263–302; 1984.

5. Dock, G. Diseases of the adrenal glands. In: Osler, W., ed. Modern medicine. Philadelphia: Lea and Febiger; 1909; 3:351–376.

6. Fehling, H. Die quantitativ Bestimmung von Zuker und Stärkmehl mittelst Kupfervitriol. Ann. d. Chem. u. Pharm. 72:106–113; 1849. Dock told the students they could use the "stomach burette" for determination of sugar by Fehling's method, but he seems to have preferred the fermentation method to the Fehling titration.

7. Directions for the tests are given in Arneill, J. R. Clinical diagnosis and urinalysis. Philadelphia: Lea Brothers and Co.; 1905:198–205.

8. Dock, G. Goitre in Michigan. Trans. Assoc. Am. Physicians 10:101–107; 1895.

9. This reason is, in fact, the fourth of Wharton's *Usus*, the first three being to remove overflow of humors from the recurrent laryngeal nerve, to warm the cartilages of the trachea, and to lubricate the larynx. See Wharton, T. Adenographia. Amsterdam: Joannis Ravensteinii; 1659:110–111.

10. Dock (n. 8).

11. Dock, G. Clinical observation in exophthalmic goitre. Am. Med. 11:271–281; 1906.

12. Magnus-Levy, A. Ueber den respiratischen Gaswechsel unter dem Einfluss der Thyroideas sowie unter verschiedenen pathologische Zuständen. Ber. klin. Wochenschr. 32:650–652; 1895.

13. Osler, W. The principles and practice of medicine. 6th ed. New York: D. Appleton and Co.; 1906:763–771. There is nothing in this section on metabolism in thyroid disease.

14. Dock, G. Diseases of the thyroid gland. In: Osler, W., ed. Modern medicine. Philadelphia: Lea and Febiger; 1909; 3:351–376.

15. Geppert, J.; Zuntz, N. Ueber die Regulation der Athmung. Arch f. d. ges. Physiol. 42:189–245; 1886.

16. Zuntz, N. Methoden den Gaswechsel zu messen. In: Hermann, L., ed. Handbuch der Physiologie. 4(2):118–129; 1882.

17. Magnus-Levy, A. Der Stoffwechsel bei Erkrankungen einiger Drüsen ohne Ausfürgang. In: von Noorden, C., ed. Handbuch der Pathologie des Stoffwechsels. Berlin: August Hirschwald; 1907; 2:311–354.

18. Magnus-Levy, A. Thyroid gland disease. In: von Noorden, C., ed. Metabolism and practical medicine. London: William Heinemann; 1907; 3:983–1017.

19. See Davenport, H. W. Physiology, 1850–1923; the view from Michigan. Bethesda, MD: American Physiological Society; 1982:68–71.

20. Dock (n. 5).

Chapter 17. Advice

1. The transcript of the informal lecture given on April 24, 1906, is heavily corrected and revised by Dock, and it served as the manuscript for an article, Dock, G. Medical ethics and etiquette. Physician and Surgeon 28:481–488; 1906. Dock hoped publication of the article would relieve him of the necessity of repeating the lecture. The last five sentences in my text are quoted from the article rather than from the transcript.

2. Rush, B. Duties of a physician. In: Runes, D. D., ed. The selected writings of Benjamin Rush. New York: Philosophical Library; 1947:308–321. Rush gave advice on how to establish and maintain a medical business. If you live in the

country, own a small farm. Grow crops, but avoid livestock; caring for the stock takes time. Go to church. Use simplicity in preparing medicines. Always appear cheerful in the presence of the patient. Perform as many autopsies as possible. Avoid consultations in plain or common cases, but ask for them in difficult and obscure ones. Etc., etc.

3. One of the editions in the Taubman Medical Library is Cathell, D. W. Book on the physician himself and things that concern his reputation and success. 10th ed. Philadelphia: F. A. Davis Co.; 1895. There was a last "Crowning Edition" in 1922. Paul Starr (The social transformation of American medicine. New York: Basic Books; 1982:86ff.) reads Cathell's detailed advice on how to make a good appearance, how to placate patients, how to foil competition and so forth as evidence of the low social status of the mass of late-nineteenth-century physicians below the thin aristocratic crust of the Bigelows, Warrens, Minots, Janeways, and Peppers.

4. Angell's handwritten draft of this letter in his file in the Bentley Historical Library is undated. If Angell's curt note is characteristic of the way Dock was treated at Michigan, it is no wonder he left.

5. Biographical details, a bibliography and full description of Hewlett's career are in Harvey, A. McG. Albion Walter Hewlett: Pioneer clinical physiologist. Johns Hopkins Med. J. 144:202–214: 1979.

6. Peterson's comments are in a letter in his file in the Bentley Historical Library.

7. Dock, G. Clinical pathology in the eighties and nineties. Am. J. Clin. Path. 16:671–680; 1946.

8. Charles C. Bass was an 1899 graduate of Tulane Medical School who began studying hookworm while practicing in Columbia, Mississippi. Soon after Dock arrived in New Orleans he collaborated with Bass in writing Hookworm disease. St. Louis: C. V. Mosby; 1910.

Index

In some instances a name is misspelled in the transcript and hence in the text, but the correct spelling is given in this index. In other instances it is not possible to distinguish between several persons with the same surname.